ANTI-INFLAMMATORY DIET 5-INGREDIENT COOKBOOK

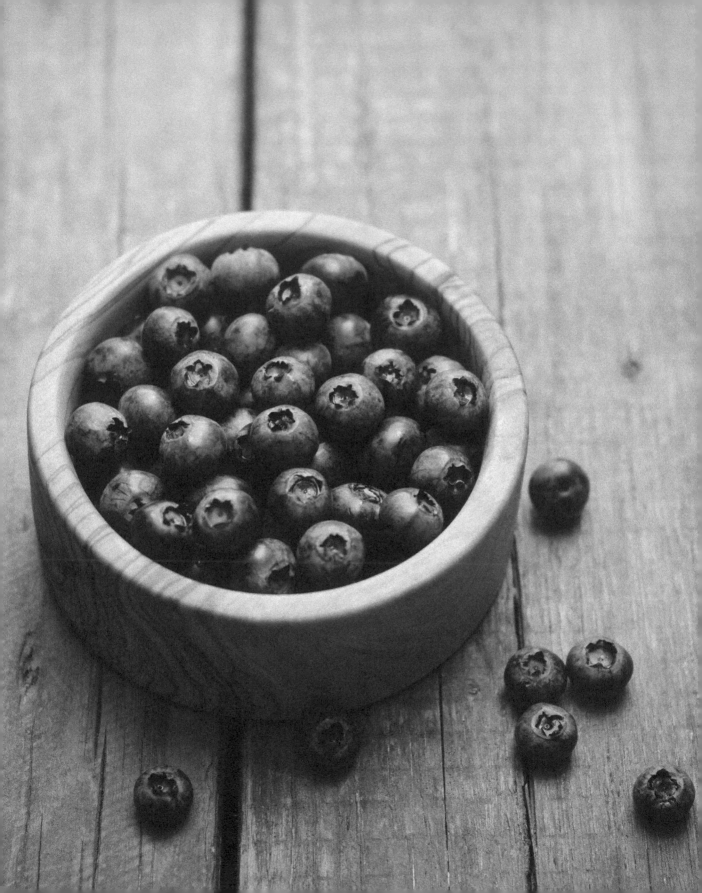

Anti-Inflammatory Diet 5-Ingredient Cookbook

FAST, EASY RECIPES TO REDUCE INFLAMMATION

NATALIE BUTLER, RDN

NUTRITION BY NATALIE

ROCKRIDGE
PRESS

Copyright © 2022 by Rockridge Press, Oakland, California

For general information on our other products and services or to obtain technical support, please contact our Customer Care Department within the United States at (866) 744-2665, or outside the United States at (510) 253-0500.

Rockridge Press publishes its books in a variety of electronic and print formats. Some content that appears in print may not be available in electronic books, and vice versa.

Some of the recipes were inspired by recipes previously published in *Anti-Inflammatory Diet in 21*, *Anti-Inflammatory Diet Meal Prep*, *Complete Anti-Inflammatory Diet for Beginners*, *Easy Anti-Inflammatory Diet*, and *One-Pot Anti-Inflammatory Cookbook*.

Interior and Cover Designer: Michael Cook
Art Producer: Megan Baggott
Editor: Anna Pulley
Production Manager: Holly Haydash

Cover photo © Antonis Achilleos. Food styling by Vanessa Desanti; Canan Czemmel/Stocksy United, ii; Jennifer Davick, x; Darren Muir, 20, 32, 58; Marta Muñoz-Calero Calderon/Stocksy United, 44; GreatStock!/StockFood USA, 78; Hélène Dujardin, 98; Ruth Black/Stocksy United, 118.

Paperback ISBN: 978-1-64876-780-7
eBook ISBN: 978-1-63807-616-2
R0

To my husband, Craig—my biggest fan,
closest confidant, best dishwasher,
and most honest taste-tester.

To my three children, Hudson, Hazel, and Holden—
your food challenges and our
evolving food journey have taught me
more than any school could.

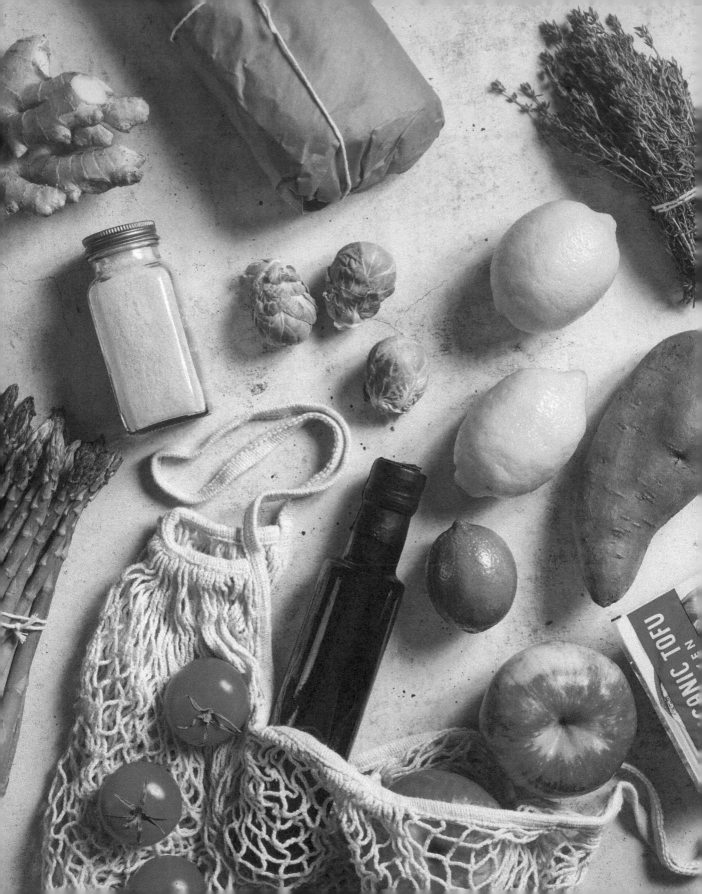

CONTENTS

INTRODUCTION ·······················

Hi! I'm Natalie Butler, RDN (Registered Dietitian Nutritionist), owner of Nutrition by Natalie, wife, and mom to three kids . . . and a whole lot of chickens! Welcome to a cookbook created for anti-inflammatory eating; recipes designed to help reduce inflammation and chronic pain, as well as improve your symptoms, lab work, omega-3 levels, and more. In other words, I'm here to help you feel better and be healthier.

My love for food goes waaaay back to childhood, but it wasn't until I took nutrition as an elective course in college (trying to help my dad feel better) that my passion was ignited. Through coursework and real-life experiences, I realized how impactful everyday food choices could be in preventing, reversing, and/or treating disease, over days, weeks, years, and a lifetime.

I understand inflammation and its destructive capabilities on both a personal and a professional level. I contracted a parasite while in college, suffered from severe postinfectious irritable bowel syndrome (IBS) afterward for years, and could tolerate only a handful of foods before I learned how to repair my gut and reduce chronic inflammation. In addition, two of my children have eosinophilic esophagitis (EoE), an inherited allergic-immune inflammatory disease of the esophagus, triggered by food and environmental allergens. I have learned firsthand how much inflammation influences their disease activity and chronic symptoms.

Inflammation is the immune process that helps an acute injury such as a scrape, a cut, a broken bone, or an infection heal. Still, it may feel temporarily uncomfortable due to redness, swelling, heat, or pain. While acute inflammation has an important, beneficial, and even healing purpose, chronic inflammation is entirely different. Chronic inflammation—which may last weeks, months, or years—can be more destructive than beneficial, leading to the damage of healthy tissue or organs and even increasing the risk of other diseases.

But there's hope. The recipes in this book will help set you on the path to healing and health. All of the recipes exclude (or significantly limit) well-known or suspected pro-inflammatory ingredients, such as processed foods, added sugars, processed meats, and trans fats, while emphasizing anti-inflammatory foods commonly found in the Mediterranean diet. Some examples include fatty fish such as salmon and sardines, walnuts, flaxseed, olive oil, eggs, cruciferous vegetables, antioxidant-rich vegetables and fruits, legumes, lean meats, and more. A Mediterranean diet is one of the most sustainable ways of eating because no major food groups are excluded, enabling you to enjoy a balanced, healthy diet and minimizing common diet-induced feelings of deprivation.

This anti-inflammatory cookbook does the hard work for you. Not only are the ingredients thoughtfully chosen, but the recipes contain only 5 or fewer main ingredients. No complicated, expensive, time-consuming recipes are coming your way. When you're dealing with chronic aches, pains, and other symptoms, the last thing you want to do is spend hours in the kitchen. Research (and my experience) shows you're less likely to be consistent with a difficult, complicated lifestyle change. So, 5-ingredient recipes save the day. Recipes in this cookbook are not only simple, healthy, and doable; they are also delicious and appeal to a variety of palates.

I have worked with thousands of patients and clients with different backgrounds, cultures, genetics, conditions, complaints, and diseases. One thing holds true across the board: Chronic inflammation does not discriminate. It underlies countless chronic diseases, including obesity, diabetes, heart disease, arthritis, and many more, and affects hundreds of millions worldwide. Inflammation will only accelerate disease progression if left uncontrolled. A proactive dietary approach is necessary to help your body heal, prevent early aging, improve symptoms, and reduce your risk of disease. This cookbook represents the passion deep in my core to help you prevent, reverse, and treat inflammation-driven disease through healthy, nutrient-dense, anti-inflammatory recipes.

Ready to feel better? Let's go!

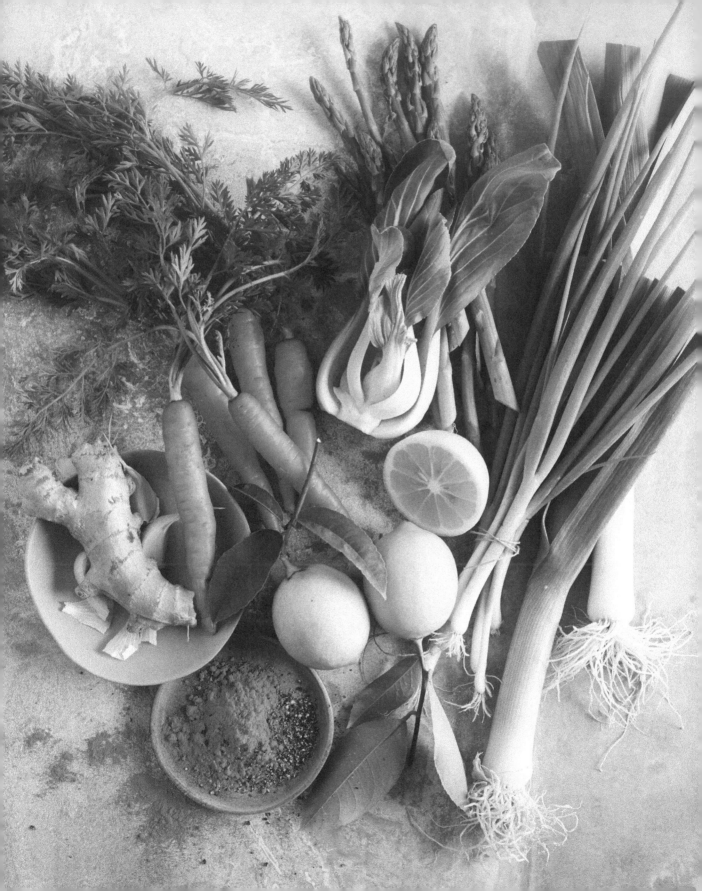

CHAPTER 1

THE 5-INGREDIENT ANTI-INFLAMMATORY SOLUTION

Chronic aches and pains and generally not feeling well are often signs of inflammation out of control. Or maybe you are one of the lucky ones and don't have daily complaints, but you see your blood sugars, weight, blood pressure, cholesterol, or other lab work worsening. I'm here to tell you that poor health doesn't have to be your fate. This chapter will give you hope. I will break down what inflammation is, why your body will do better with less, and everything you need to know about eating an anti-inflammatory diet.

WHAT IS INFLAMMATION?

When the immune system is working properly, inflammation plays an important role in our body's healthy response to injury or infection. Our immune system rallies to restore health upon injury or infection, such as a scrape on the knee or exposure to the cold everyone else has at the office. This leads to a period of acute inflammation, which promotes healing as the body's defensive process repairs and restores integrity. Once the problem is successfully managed, the immune response downregulates and the inflammation around the area of injury or infection subsides.

When you notice that a paper cut on your finger is red, swollen, warm, and painful, this is all part of inflammation, which is taking place because of a smoothly running immune system. Immune cells are activated to the site of the problem, so blood flow in the area increases, leading to the experience of swelling and heat, which will subside as the wound heals. Soon you'll have nothing to remember the paper cut by but a thin line of scar tissue. This kind of acute, localized inflammation may not require any additional treatment; however, maintaining a consistent anti-inflammatory diet such as the one described in this book will ensure that your body has all the nutrients needed to support even a minor healing process.

Conversely, a little cut that seems to hang on too long, remaining puffy and painful, and not making much progress in healing might indicate a bigger issue. In this case, the normal process of acute inflammation may have continued unchecked, signaling an underlying chronic inflammation that is more problematic. This can occur because of an unhealed infection such as hepatitis B or C, prolonged exposure to environmental toxins such as cigarette smoke, or existing health conditions such as obesity or autoimmune disease. Lifestyle factors such as diet and stress can also amplify the inflammatory response. At first, there may not be any obvious symptoms of this kind of ongoing low-grade inflammation. Yet, in the long term, chronic inflammation can increase the risk for or exacerbate various health problems.

Conditions Related to Excessive Inflammation

Recent research has linked chronic inflammation to a wide range of diseases and health conditions, including:

- Crohn's disease
- Heart/cardiovascular disease
- Hypertension
- Inflammatory bowel disease
- Metabolic syndrome
- Nonalcoholic fatty liver disease
- Obesity
- Pancreatitis
- Rheumatoid arthritis
- Some cancers—especially colorectal, gastric, esophageal, pancreatic, breast, endometrial, and ovarian
- Type 2 diabetes
- Ulcerative colitis

Chronic inflammation can cause, exacerbate, or result from these types of health conditions. Repeated or unchecked inflammatory responses play a role in the many complex biological pathways by which disease may result or be worsened. In these disease pathways, protein messengers called *cytokines* are released as part of the immune response. Some cytokines participate in your body's defensive response to a health threat and accelerate the inflammatory response, while others are anti-inflammatory and help restore balance as you heal. If the balance of pro-inflammatory to anti-inflammatory cytokines is disrupted, normal cell function can be impaired, and health and well-being may suffer. It can be hard to tell which came first: the inflammation or the health condition to which it is linked.

With obesity, for example, a series of causes and effects interact with each other in a downward spiral of declining health. Chronic, low-grade inflammation results directly from the consumption of excess calories, high blood sugar, and obesity. As fat tissue increases, it releases chemicals, hormones, and immune cells that can disrupt normal body function. Pro-inflammatory cytokines are also released, leading to higher levels of inflammation throughout the body. As the internal system becomes more imbalanced, the risk of developing chronic disorders or diseases such as cardiovascular disease, hypertension, type 2 diabetes, and various cancers increases. Many of these conditions increase inflammation themselves. It can become complicated when so many of the body's systems are poorly regulated and caught in a negative feedback loop of active inflammation and damage to other systems.

But there's good news: Consuming anti-inflammatory foods can help straighten out the whole situation, whatever it may be rooted in. An anti-inflammatory diet can support healing if inflammation already exists, and it will provide a foundation for resilience in the future. Shift your focus to this kind of nourishing, balanced, and tasty diet, and you'll see the difference, as this way of eating will restore the energy and sense of well-being you long for.

Anti-Inflammatory Diet Basics

Experts agree that a diet consisting of a wide range of plant-based foods, accompanied by moderate amounts of fibrous whole grains, lean proteins, and healthy fats, is the type of eating pattern that will reduce inflammation and ensure a robust and balanced immune system. We are constantly learning more about the negative effects of heavily processed, packaged foods, which are often high in inflammation-promoting sodium, added sugars, refined grains, and detrimental fats. Conversely, this book emphasizes fresh, whole foods that are prepared using healthy cooking techniques. Vibrant herbs and spices are not just good for punching up flavor—you'll also learn how each brings its own health-supportive qualities to your meals. Prebiotic and probiotic foods support your microbiome—that's the name for the beneficial gut bacteria in your digestive system. These bacteria are linked to a thriving immune system. And you can wash it all down with powerful inflammation-fighting beverages such as unsweetened tea and coffee, water infused with herbs or fruit, and the occasional glass of red wine, if you choose to partake.

I present recipes inspired by the many traditional cuisines around the world that promote a vigorous immune response. Traditional Japanese diets, for instance, are low in fat and full of nutrient-rich vegetables and seafood but contain very little sugar or refined flour. A modified paleo approach is also explored here, including generous portions of vegetables and hearty dishes prepared from the healthiest proteins. The Mediterranean eating pattern is well studied for its anti-inflammatory, health-promoting qualities, and many people find its flavors satisfying and appealing. It is based on abundant fruits and vegetables, along with whole grains, legumes, and nuts. Fish, red wine, and olive oil are incorporated regularly in Mediterranean cooking, while red meat, added sugars, and high-fat dairy are limited. This delicious eating style inspires me, so you'll see many recipes here that reflect the Mediterranean approach. But I also recognize that the only anti-inflammatory diet that will work for you is the one you find satisfying and delicious and that avoids your individual food triggers. So, after you master the basics, use these principles to figure out which styles you enjoy best and fine-tune your own anti-inflammatory lifestyle path.

HOW AN ANTI-INFLAMMATORY DIET HELPS HEAL

There is a direct link between food and inflammation. A study published in the *Journal of Internal Medicine* found that foods naturally containing antioxidants can reduce inflammation in the body and damage from free radicals. *Free radicals* are highly reactive molecules with one or more unpaired electrons. When the body has an overload of free radicals, it can enter a state of oxidative stress, and they can begin to damage DNA and healthy cells in the body. Some research, including a study published in *Current Opinion in Food Science*, has indicated that the oxidative stress caused by free radicals can be stabilized by antioxidants found in the food you eat. For example, the antioxidant vitamin C, found in broccoli, bell peppers, berries, and citrus, gives its electrons to free radicals in the body, helping prevent damage and leading to reduced inflammation.

There's something special about the anti-inflammatory properties of whole foods. Every fruit, vegetable, grain, and legume has a food matrix: the unique, complex structure of the whole food. An apple, for example, contains water, fiber, and a large variety of vitamins, minerals, and antioxidants. If you juice, dry, or even grind the apple up into pills, you're altering the food matrix and changing how the apple interacts with the body. This book focuses on preparing food to remain as close as possible to its whole, unprocessed form.

Foods that Heal

Many foods contain potent anti-inflammatory properties. These include whole grains, legumes, citrus and other fruits and berries, nuts and chia seeds, cocoa, teas, and herbs and spices such as ginger, turmeric, and garlic.

Cocoa. Chocolate, specifically antioxidant-rich, over 70 percent cocoa, has been shown to have anti-inflammatory properties, according to research published in *Nutrients* and other journals. It's important to incorporate pure dark chocolate more often, rather than prepared chocolate with added sugars and dairy. Include cocoa in your diet three to four times per week.

Fruits and vegetables. Fruits and vegetables are rich in a variety of antioxidants, including vitamins C and E. The Dietary Guidelines for Americans recommend making them the central part of your diet. According to recent data from the Centers for Disease Control and Prevention, only 12.2 percent and 9.3 percent of Americans currently meet their fruit and vegetable intake recommendations, respectively. The different colors of fruits, berries, and vegetables indicate different types of antioxidants. You may have heard the advice to "eat the rainbow," which refers to eating a wide variety of foods to fill the body with different healthy compounds. Include at least 5 servings of fruit and vegetables in your diet per day, with the majority being vegetables.

Herbs, spices, and tea. Herbs and spices are a vital part of an anti-inflammatory diet. Garlic, cinnamon, and turmeric should be staples in your pantry. Ginger is an herb that has been specifically associated with calming inflammation. Not only does it soothe the stomach and reduce nausea, but studies, including one published in the *Journal of Medicinal Food*, have shown that it can significantly reduce levels of CRP (C-reactive protein, a protein sent to the bloodstream in response to inflammation). Tea (especially green and black) is another antioxidant-rich ingredient that has been shown to calm inflammation in the body, according to research published in *Brain, Behavior, and Immunity*. Incorporate herbs, spices, and tea multiple times per day into your diet.

Legumes. Beans, lentils, and soy foods have been linked with reduced inflammation in many studies, including ones published in *Nutrition*. They are rich in fiber (3 to 4 times higher than brown rice), vitamins, minerals, and many antioxidants. Legumes contain a balance of protein and complex carbohydrates, so they're filling, and they'll fuel your energy production. Eating whole and fermented soy foods, such as tofu, tempeh, miso, and edamame, may reduce inflammation in the body due to their high fiber and antioxidant content. The current Dietary Guidelines for Americans and the American Institute for Cancer Research suggest that soy foods may benefit the cardiovascular system and bone health and may even help prevent some cancers. If you have a digestive disorder such as gastroparesis or irritable bowel syndrome, the legume family may need to be limited or excluded, at least temporarily, for you to feel your best. For others, I recommend a serving of legumes at least once per day in your diet.

Nuts, seeds, and omega-3s. Nuts and seeds contain many important anti-inflammatory nutrients, including antioxidant vitamin E and heart-healthy unsaturated fatty acids. Some nuts and seeds, such as chia, flax, and walnuts, contain a unique healthy fat called omega-3 fatty acids. According to research in the *American Journal of Clinical Nutrition* and other journals, omega-3s have been shown to reduce inflammation in the body. Cold-water fish such as salmon and halibut are another source of omega-3s. Include a portion of nuts and seeds daily and omega-3-rich fish at least three times per week into your diet.

Whole grains. High-fiber whole grains, including oats, wild rice, and quinoa (which is actually a seed), are packed with vitamins, minerals, and antioxidants. According to research published in *Nutrition Reviews*, consuming whole grains (as opposed to processed "white" flour products such as white bread, pastries, and cookies) could lower inflammatory markers in the body, including CRP. Some people are allergic to or intolerant of wheat or gluten (a protein in wheat, spelt, farro, bulgur, and semolina—used to make pasta—which can accelerate inflammation if consumed). Because of this, almost all the recipes in this book will emphasize gluten-free grains. Include a serving of whole grains (or nutrient-rich alternatives like legumes) at least once per day in your diet.

THE ANTI-INFLAMMATORY DIET AT A GLANCE

FOODS TO INCLUDE	FOODS TO LIMIT OR AVOID
Allium family (garlic, scallions, onions, shallots)	Artificial sweeteners
All herbs and spices, particularly ginger, turmeric, cinnamon	Dairy (full-fat and high-lactose milk, cream, butter, cheese, yogurt)
All vegetables except nightshades, only if intolerant (see next column)	Fried foods
Avocados	Margarine
Coffee, low to moderate intake	Nightshade vegetables (tomatoes, white potatoes, eggplant, peppers, goji berries)
Dark chocolate	Oils (vegetable, soybean, canola, coconut)
Eggs	Processed meats (bacon, sausage, deli meats, hot dogs)
Fermented foods such as kimchi, kombucha, and sauerkraut	Refined carbohydrates (breakfast cereals, desserts)
Fish (especially wild-caught salmon, sardines, mackerel, anchovies, herring)	Soda and other sugar-sweetened beverages
Fruit, especially berries	Sweeteners (sugar, high-fructose corn syrup, agave syrup, and candy)
Gluten-free grains (buckwheat, millet, oats, quinoa, rice, wild rice)	Wheat and grains containing gluten (bread, pasta, wheat-based cereals, rye, barley)
Gluten-free high-fiber pasta	
Grass-fed beef	
Honey, maple syrup	
Legumes (beans and lentils)	

FOODS TO INCLUDE	FOODS TO LIMIT OR AVOID
Nuts and seeds, excluding peanuts	
Oils (olive, avocado, flax, walnut, olive oil, MCT)	
Poultry	
Soy products, including tofu	
Sweet potatoes	
Tea (green and black)	

Drinking Enough Water

The body relies on getting enough water to work properly. Water helps regulate energy levels and is critical for brain function, skin integrity, and mood. Water makes up most of your blood volume, where it helps transport nutrients from the food you eat to the tissues that need it. Water helps detoxify the body, removing waste through sweat, urine, and bowel movements. The National Academy of Medicine (formerly called the Institute of Medicine) has set guidelines for total water intake at 2.7 liters per day (about 92 ounces) for adult females and 3.7 liters per day (about 126 ounces) for adult males. These amounts include water in liquid form as well as water present in foods. Not meeting your fluid needs may cause headaches and/or constipation, increase the risk of kidney stones and even impair attention and cognition. When planning your weekly meals, make sure that you set water-intake goals. Fill a pitcher of water and keep it in your refrigerator or on your counter to keep it at the front of your mind. Purchase a reusable water bottle and set goals for how many times you need to refill it daily. You can also try infusing your water with fruit, vegetables, or herbs for more flavor and anti-inflammatory support.

Foods to Limit or Avoid

I might as well get the difficult news out of the way: There are foods you need to avoid or significantly limit to help reduce inflammation. I don't enjoy restricting people's diets, but in some cases, it is necessary. So let's dive in.

Certain fats and oils. Canola oil, vegetable oils, trans fats, and margarine may trigger inflammation. Vegetable oils and margarine are high in omega-6 fats, which can be inflammatory at high levels, especially when they are out of balance with anti-inflammatory omega-3 fats. Canola oil should be avoided due to the way it is made—the high-heat process can cause the oil to become rancid and inflammatory.

While some trans fats are present in natural foods, the majority of trans fats are manufactured fats that adversely affect cardiovascular disease and other risk factors because of their highly inflammatory properties. Trans fats are primarily found in processed foods and fried foods. Due to recent bans in the United States and other countries, artificial trans fats must be eliminated from all processed foods in their respective countries; therefore, added trans fats are less of a concern.

Certain fruits and vegetables. Most fruits and vegetables are anti-inflammatory and should be the basis of any healthy diet. The exception, for some people with specific food sensitivities, is nightshades. Intolerance, however, is not nearly as common as generally believed, and research shows many nightshades are indeed anti-inflammatory.

One thing to note about fruit: Although it is highly nutritious, some fruits are lower in nutrients and higher in sugar, which may increase insulin. High levels of circulating insulin and blood sugar are pro-inflammatory. Sugar sensitivity can vary from person to person. If you are sensitive to sugar, avoid eating excessive fruit, especially low-fiber fruits such as tropical fruits and grapes. One to two servings per day is enough to meet your nutrient needs and give you a little sweet treat.

Dairy. The evidence on dairy and inflammation is inconsistent, but dairy is a common food intolerance for many people due to the milk sugar lactose. Lactose intolerance is one of the most common food intolerances in the world. Dairy proteins, not lactose, are also the top food allergen in children worldwide. A review of 52 studies on dairy and inflammation in *Critical Reviews in Food Science and*

Nutrition found that dairy was inflammatory for those who could not tolerate it or have an allergy.

Once again, whether you need to avoid dairy comes down to individual tolerance. Symptoms of lactose intolerance include gas, bloating, diarrhea, or other digestive problems. Lactose-intolerance symptoms are generally more severe with liquid milk, while small amounts of cheese or yogurt can frequently be tolerated.

Because lactose intolerance is quite common, there are no recipes that include high-lactose cow's milk or cream in this book. There is one recipe using sheep's or goat's milk, as those tend to be better tolerated by most people.

Gluten. Wheat (and rye and barley) contain a protein called *gluten*, which is a major trigger for inflammation. Limit wheat and foods made from wheat, though it is important to rule out celiac disease before going gluten-free; otherwise, you may receive false-negative test results. Foods containing gluten may include breads, cereals, pasta, cakes, cookies, pies, and other desserts.

Certain compounds in gluten can damage the digestive system lining, leading to a condition called intestinal permeability or "leaky gut." When the gut is "leaky," it allows too many food particles, microbes, and other substances to pass through without proper digestion. This causes the immune system to react to these substances, leading to dysfunction or inflammation. Avoiding foods containing gluten allows the gut to heal, a major step toward controlling inflammation. It is important to choose naturally gluten-free whole foods to obtain enough fiber for gut bacteria and healthy bowel function, rather than relying on processed gluten-free versions of foods.

For some, reintroduction of gluten-containing foods is tolerated, and consumption of low intakes of gluten can be maintained long-term with minimal impact on inflammation. For others, long-term avoidance is ideal. I recommend pre- and post-intervention lab work and working with a dietitian to help with this process.

Processed meat. As much as meat is blamed for all the ills in the world, poultry, eggs, and fish are not inflammatory foods. You will see these on the "Foods to Include" table on page 8. However, processed meats, such as bacon, sausage, deli meats, and hot dogs, may worsen inflammation. These meats are also linked to an increased risk of diabetes, heart disease, and stroke. The reason is that they are higher in compounds called *advanced glycation end products* and *saturated fats*, which are known to cause inflammation. Avoid or limit processed meats as much as possible.

Other inflammatory no-nos. Food high in sugar should also be avoided or significantly limited. Candy, cookies, pies, cakes, sweetened beverages, and even artificial sweeteners can trigger inflammation. Excessive sugar intake has been linked with an increased risk of inflammatory and chronic diseases.

The *World Journal of Gastroenterology* states that alcohol has been shown to be inflammatory in those who are not healthy and can perpetuate existing systemic inflammation through an increase in cytokines and the toxic bacterial product lipopolysaccharide (LPS). Avoid or significantly limit alcohol of all kinds if you are struggling with severe inflammation.

GETTING STARTED WITH THE ANTI-INFLAMMATORY DIET

Here are my top tips to help you transition to an anti-inflammatory diet. Simple swaps to add healthy fats and prioritizing fruits and vegetables can greatly affect inflammation in the body.

Increase foods you enjoy. Adapting to an anti-inflammatory diet shouldn't require turning your world upside down. Focus on increasing the anti-inflammatory foods you already enjoy, and the other foods will fall away naturally.

Keep an open mind. Try new foods and prepare foods you didn't previously enjoy in new ways. There's no need to eat plain, unseasoned vegetables, beans, or grains—the herbs and spices used in these recipes will help maximize flavor.

Meet your own needs and preferences. The recipes in this book are meant to be flexible. If you have specific food allergies or preferences, adjust to suit your needs. I'll offer substitutions and tips along the way so that you can adapt easily.

Swap in healthy fats. Cook with fats and oils that come from natural sources. Use fats such as olive oil and avocado oil and add plenty of omega-3-rich ingredients, such as chia and flax seeds, walnuts, and fatty fish.

Rethink snacks. Simplify your snack options by choosing fruits, vegetables, nuts and seeds, and homemade dips and spreads. This book includes many easy-to-make and packable snacks, so there's no need to purchase packaged chips or crackers.

Include fruits and vegetables in every meal. In an anti-inflammatory diet plan, your meals will revolve around produce. Stocking up on fresh and frozen fruits and vegetables will help you include them in every meal and snack so you can meet your daily goals with ease.

Healthy Eating for Everyone

Whether or not you have chronic inflammation, eating an anti-inflammatory diet can benefit your health. This is because an anti-inflammatory diet is made up of healthy foods. It maximizes nutrient-dense foods full of fiber, vitamins, minerals, and antioxidants. For this reason, an anti-inflammatory diet can benefit people of all ages with all types of health needs.

If you do experience chronic inflammation in the body and are suffering from associated diseases or fatigue, the anti-inflammatory diet can change your life. You may see your test results for CRP or other inflammatory markers improve. You may notice improved energy levels, have less chronic pain, experience fewer symptom flare-ups, and sleep more peacefully. You may find you can resume doing things you loved but had to give up.

As you grow accustomed to eating anti-inflammatory foods, you may feel it become easy and effortless. You might feel more in control of your schedule and feel positive about what you're putting in your body. I recommend trying this dietary eating plan for 4 to 6 weeks and tracking your symptoms, followed by repeat labs, so you can get a better idea of the changes you experience.

Small Lifestyle Changes

A healthy diet is essential to feel your best, but if you pair the healthiest diet with an unhealthy lifestyle, you risk stalling your progress. Work with your body, not against it, by practicing healthy lifestyle choices each day.

Exercise: Exercise isn't limited to a gym. Walking, hiking, dancing, swimming, and biking all count. Find something you enjoy and make that your foundation. Aim for light- to moderate-intensity exercise or infrequent short bouts of intense exercise, rather than prolonged, intense exercise, for the most benefits.

Reduce toxin exposure: *Obesogens* are chemicals in your environment (in toys, cookware, plastics, and cosmetics) that can interfere with metabolism and may increase hunger, enlarge fat cells, reduce calorie burn, and increase CRP. Smoke, BPA, parabens, phthalates, and pesticides are just a few to avoid. I recommend the use of stainless steel pans, glass containers (rather than plastic), and nontoxic health and beauty and cleaning products.

Sleep: Sleep is when your body repairs, heals, reduces cortisol (your primary stress hormone), cleanses the brain and intestines, and defends against chronic inflammation. Sleep disturbance, poor sleep quality, and short sleep duration are linked with inflammatory disease risk, mortality, and increased CRP and interleukin-6 (IL-6). Aim for 7 to 9 hours of quality sleep in a dark, cold room every night, and avoid eating and exposure to blue light from screens for several hours before bed.

Reduce stress: Chronic stress over-activates the nervous system, resulting in higher circulating levels of stress hormones, leading to a pro-inflammatory state and a compromised immune system. Deep breathing, meditation, exercise, and time in nature can improve how the body handles stressors.

Timing meals and fasting: Nutrition and health isn't just *what* you eat, but *when* you eat, too. Shortening your daily eating window to 8 to 12 hours (and fasting the other hours) can help reduce common drivers of inflammation-driving weight gain and obesity like overconsumption of calories and eating late at night.

THE 5-INGREDIENT SOLUTION

Gone are the days of hours in the kitchen, tedious preparation of long ingredient lists, and laborious cooking to eat healthy. No need to surrender to takeout or endless leftovers, either. My 5-ingredient solution comes to the rescue: This cookbook's philosophy hinges on recipes with no more than 5 ingredients (excluding such "freebies" as water, salt, pepper, and olive oil—see page 16), the perfect solution for anyone battling inflammation, aches and pains, and chronic symptoms. Every 5-ingredient recipe has been created with the fundamental goal to help you feel better, with more ease. Here are five reasons why you'll love 5-ingredient recipes and why they'll love you back.

1. **No more guessing games; you know what you're eating.** Not sure what foods bother you or help you feel better? Had a flare-up from a meal but have no idea what caused it? Simple recipes with limited ingredients will help you quickly identify what foods are best for your body.

2. **Easy to follow and stick to.** A major reason diets or lifestyle changes fail is a lack of consistency. When motivation is strong—often during the first few weeks of change—anything seems possible. When motivation wanes or life throws a curveball, difficult tasks or those that require lots of attention or effort get pushed to the back burner. Easy recipes mean you'll be able to be consistent with prioritizing your health.

3. **Fresh, whole foods.** Clean eating with fresh, whole foods means your body is receiving nutrient density with every bite, not filling up on processed, inflammatory calories. The ingredients in this book are chosen carefully to give you the most benefit from each recipe. With whole foods, your body gets the antioxidants, phytochemicals, vitamins, minerals, fiber, and anti-inflammatory fats it desperately craves to feel better. Plus, you'll minimize symptoms from any unknown intolerances to the food additives, preservatives, emulsifiers, and flavor enhancers found in processed foods.

4. **Time and budget-friendly.** Five-ingredient recipes respect your time by freeing you up in the kitchen quicker to focus on other essential tasks such as family time, exercise, relaxation, self-care, and more. In addition, a shorter ingredient list means fewer trips to the grocery store, which is easier on the wallet.

5. **Less daunting and feels empowering.** Ever delayed trying something new because it felt too overwhelming to tackle? Simple and easy recipes make changing your eating approachable, achievable, and doable. No long, difficult recipes in sight; no master chef skills required. You'll feel empowered with 85 simple recipes under your belt.

Simple Staples

While we hold firm to our 5-ingredient rule for recipes, we aren't counting the following essential pantry staples. Don't have these on hand? Stock up on your next grocery trip.

Olive oil: Olive oil is a staple in the Mediterranean diet, a well-researched diet for health and longevity. Olive oil's benefits stem from its polyphenols, oleic acid, and phytosterols. I recommend extra-virgin olive oil for the most anti-inflammatory benefits, but for high-heat cooking, refined olive oil or avocado oil is best. A good-quality olive oil is stored in a dark, glass jar and has an almost spicy or peppery aftertaste.

Salt and black pepper: When used in the correct amounts in recipes, salt should heighten the flavors of individual ingredients without tasting overwhelmingly salty. Salt—a significant source of sodium—is added in low to moderate amounts in my recipes because it may be pro-inflammatory for some. Black pepper, which adds a mild spice and depth of flavor, also has antibacterial, antioxidant, and anti-inflammatory benefits.

Anti-Inflammatory Supermarket Shortcuts

Peeled or cooked shrimp. Peeling shrimp can be such a fiddly task; spend a little extra money and buy them peeled. Cooked shrimp are a great addition to a dinner salad.

Canned fish. Though fresh fish cooks quickly, canned fish is shelf-stable, doesn't require any cooking time, and can be eaten plain or as a simple ingredient in other meals.

Cubed winter squash. Cutting and peeling a raw squash can be tough. Cubed (frozen or fresh) winter squash significantly reduces prep time.

Frozen vegetable mixes. Make it easy to sneak a ton of vegetables into various dishes with little prep.

Mashed avocado. Prepping avocados adds time to your recipe. Go for mashed or guacamole to speed up the process. They tend to last a bit longer mashed in a prepackaged container.

Pineapple slices. Peeling and cutting a pineapple can be cumbersome, so let someone else handle it.

Premade kebabs. Someone else has already taken care of prepping the meat and vegetables; now all you do is cook them.

Pre-marinated meats. For nights when you can't even think about what to make, these are quick and easy to prepare. (Check the ingredients in the marinade, because they may include soy sauce [which contains gluten] and sugar.)

Preportioned or bulk nuts. Nuts are a great healthy snack; preportioning helps you take them on the go. Bulk nuts can be stored in the freezer and removed as needed.

Rotisserie chicken. Makes for a quick weekday lunch, or it can be shredded into soups or salad for added protein. (Check the ingredients in the seasonings, because they may include sugar.)

Steamer bags. Whether fresh or frozen, steamer bags of vegetables are washed and prepped, reducing your time in the kitchen. Also, many can be eaten raw without cooking.

Helpful Kitchen Gadgets

Some kitchen gadgets can come in handy when you want to eat healthy but have reduced energy and/or time. Produce prep is one of the lengthiest parts of cooking and may prevent people from eating more fruits and vegetables. The gadgets below are inexpensive yet worth their weight in gold for simplifying your food prep and cooking process.

Blender. This is one of my most-used items. I don't just use it for smoothies, either. If you purchase a high-power version, no job is too much. Juice fruits and vegetables, create sauces, crush ice, chop onions, make soups, blend oat flour, or make nut milk. You can even minimize muffin cleanup by making muffin batter in a blender.

Cast-iron skillet. This is a sturdy nonstick pan that can be used on the stovetop or in the oven. It's easy to clean and cuts down on the number of pans that get dirty. I often use a large cast-iron skillet to make multiple protein servings at one time or cook a one-pan meal including both protein and vegetables.

Citrus juicer. Hand-squeezing lemons, limes, or oranges is an option. But when you need more than ¼ cup of juice in a recipe or want to jazz up water or tea, a citrus juicer speeds up the process while removing pesky seeds.

Food chopper/slicer. I recommend choosing a gadget with multiple functions for limited budgets. A freestanding grater used for cheese can do so much more than that. Grate zucchini, slice radishes, or mince garlic. A mandoline is the epitome of a useful gadget, slicing soft and tough vegetables in record time with minimal cleanup. Other handy gadgets in this category include a manual food chopper and zester.

Food processor. Processors have wider bases than blenders, so they work better to mince, puree, and chop dry and/or thick ingredients. Small processors are excellent for quickly mincing a batch of garlic cloves, fresh herbs, hot peppers, or for creating a quick sauce. A large processor is ideal to create a large volume of a recipe—bulk batching—to be enjoyed now and later. Hummus and finely grating or slicing carrots and squash are some of my frequent uses for the processor.

Garlic press. A garlic press is a handheld tool used specifically to mince peeled, raw garlic cloves quickly and efficiently. Garlic is used throughout the recipes in this cookbook, so this is a wonderful tool to have at your disposal.

ABOUT THE RECIPES

I designed the recipes in this cookbook to be simple, healthy, and reduce inflammation. The recipes avoid pro-inflammatory ingredients while including healing, nutrient-rich, and anti-inflammatory ingredients. Recipes exclude omega-6-rich foods and ingredients such as soybean and vegetable oils, peanuts, trans fats, added refined sugars, refined grains, and pastries, and they also limit high amounts of saturated fat.

Tips

I provide tips on most of the recipes to enable you to customize and/or reduce your time in the kitchen. The prep tip shows how to speed up prep or the cooking process, or to accomplish the recipe in an easier way. The variation tip offers substitutions or additions to modify the flavor, texture, or nutrition.

Labels

Dairy-Free: Dairy can be high in saturated fat which can cause inflammation. It also contains proteins which are allergens, and lactose (sugars) that are not tolerated by many worldwide.

Gluten-Free: Avoids wheat, rye, and barley, as well as condiments and prepared foods that commonly contain gluten. Be sure to read product labels to ensure that they are certified gluten-free and produced in a facility where there is no risk of cross-contamination.

No Added Sugar: These have no added sugar and may rely on small amounts of natural sweeteners such as honey or sweet fruits.

Nut-Free: While peanuts are technically a legume, any tree nut or peanuts are excluded in the recipe if it carries this label.

Omega-3-Rich: These contain higher amounts of anti-inflammatory fats such as fatty fish, eggs, walnuts, flaxseed, and more.

Soy-Free: Excludes all forms of soy, including soy milk, edamame, tofu, soy sauce, miso, soy protein isolate, and soybean oil.

Vegan: Avoids all animal products, such as meat, dairy, eggs, and honey.

Vegetarian: Excludes meat but may still contain dairy, eggs, and/or honey.

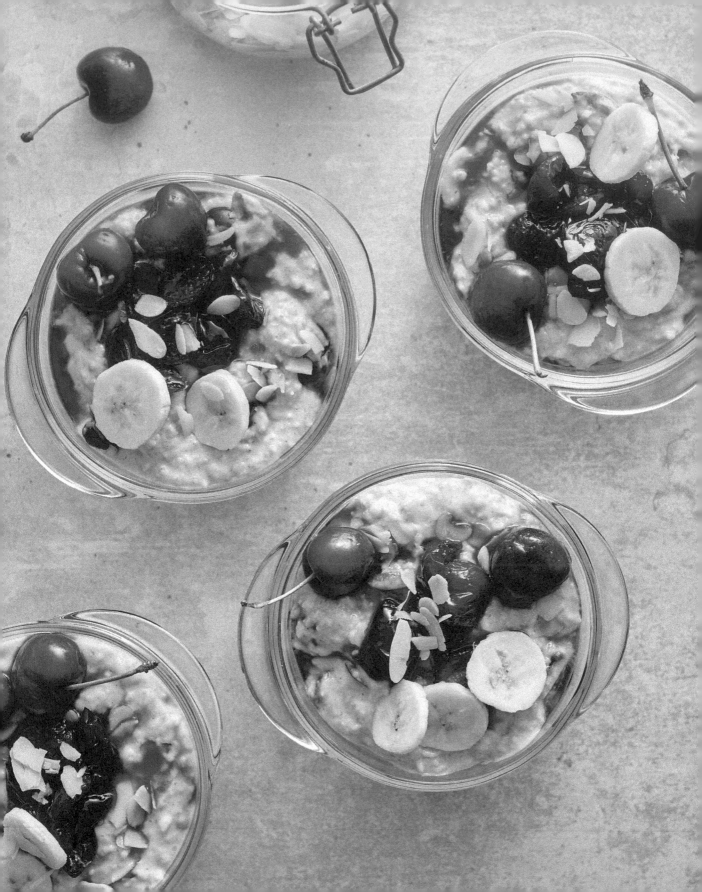

CHAPTER 2

BREAKFAST

Sweet Potato Toast

Gluten-Free, Omega-3-Rich, No Added Sugar, Nut-Free, Soy-Free, Vegetarian
Prep time: 5 minutes / **Cook time:** 10 minutes • **Serves** 4

Sweet potato toast is a wonderful alternative to traditional gluten-containing toast. This recipe boasts anti-inflammatory carotenoids in the sweet potato and spinach, both complemented by the smoky and spicy flavor of the chipotle yogurt sauce. Choose eggs from pastured hens for a higher level of anti-inflammatory omega-3s.

2 medium sweet potatoes, washed and cut into ¼-inch-thick slices

2 tablespoons extra-virgin olive oil, divided

3 or 4 chipotle peppers in adobo (from a 7.5-ounce can), plus more as needed

1 cup low-fat or nonfat Greek yogurt

1 cup fresh spinach, torn or chopped

8 large eggs, fried or poached

1. Lightly brush each side of each slice of sweet potato with olive oil.

2. In a toaster or toaster oven on a medium-high setting, toast the slices. Cook them for 2 to 3 cycles, or until soft.

3. Put 3 to 4 chipotle peppers in a food processor and pulse to mince. Alternatively, you may mince the peppers by hand. Reserve the can contents.

4. Add the yogurt to the food processor bowl (or use a separate bowl if mincing by hand). Stir to combine. Taste and add more peppers or a tablespoon of the sauce from the can to increase the spice level.

5. To serve, plate the sweet potato slices and top with 1 tablespoon of sauce, about ¼ cup of spinach, 1 egg, and another 1 tablespoon of sauce on top.

PREP TIP: To make this recipe for a crowd, bake the sweet potato slices in a 400°F oven for 5 to 10 minutes. Check for doneness by piercing with a fork; they should be soft.

Per Serving (2 slices): Calories: 312; Total fat: 17g; Saturated fat: 5g; Sodium: 229mg; Carbohydrates: 21g; Fiber: 3g; Sugar: 9g; Protein: 18g

Loaded Almond Butter and Avocado Toast

Dairy-Free, Soy-Free, Vegetarian
Prep time: 2 minutes / **Cook time:** 2 minutes • **Serves 2**

You might not have seen this combination before, but this loaded toast is packed with healthy fats and will satisfy your palate and your hunger. It's a favorite meal in my household, even for the kids. Choosing a higher-fiber bread—greater than 3 grams of fiber per slice—will not only nourish gut bacteria but will also keep your blood sugar more stable, especially when combined with the avocado and almond butter.

2 slices whole-grain bread or gluten-free
  bread, toasted
¼ cup almond butter
1 avocado, pitted, peeled, and sliced

2 teaspoons honey
Red pepper flakes
Sea salt

On each slice of toast, layer 2 tablespoons almond butter and half the avocado. Drizzle 1 teaspoon of honey on top and sprinkle with red pepper flakes and salt.

VARIATION TIP: For a nut-free option, simply replace the almond butter with sunflower seed or pumpkin seed butter. For a gluten-free option, choose a gluten-free bread or even Sweet Potato Toast (page 22).

Per Serving: Calories: 443; Total fat: 33g; Saturated fat: 4g; Sodium: 186mg; Carbohydrates: 32g; Fiber: 12g; Sugar: 10g; Protein: 12g

Spicy Turmeric Egg Scramble

Gluten-Free, No Added Sugar, Omega-3-Rich, Soy-Free, Vegetarian
Prep time: 10 minutes / **Cook time:** 10 minutes • **Serves** 2

These aren't boring scrambled eggs. Garlic is a nutritional powerhouse—it's anti-bacterial, antiviral, antioxidant-rich, anti-inflammatory, and more. Choose fresh garlic, rather than a peeled or jarred option, for these benefits. Pro tip: Allow the minced garlic to rest 10 minutes before cooking or consuming to enable the beneficial sulfur compound allicin to multiply. To obtain the most health benefits from garlic, it's best to eat it uncooked or lightly cooked more often than well-cooked. Cottage cheese is a salted cheese, so you can likely skip adding extra salt to this recipe.

2 teaspoons extra-virgin olive oil

4 large eggs, whisked

½ cup low-fat cottage cheese

2 garlic cloves, freshly minced and set aside for 10 minutes

½ teaspoon ground turmeric

¼ teaspoon cayenne pepper

1. In a medium nonstick skillet, heat the olive oil over medium heat.

2. Add the eggs and cottage cheese and whisk to combine. Add the garlic, turmeric, and cayenne pepper, and whisk again. Cook for 3 to 5 minutes, gently stirring occasionally to prevent browning on the bottom.

3. When the eggs are set (liquid is mostly absorbed), remove the skillet from the heat. Sprinkle more pepper, if desired, and serve warm.

VARIATION TIP: This is a versatile recipe that is ideal for cleaning out your produce drawer. You can add 1 cup dark leafy greens, onion, or bell pepper remnants to boost the nutrition. Simply sauté the vegetables in step 1 but before adding the eggs in step 2. Add the eggs when the vegetables soften, usually after 3 to 4 minutes of cooking.

Per Serving: Calories: 231; Total fat: 15g; Saturated fat: 4g; Sodium: 372mg; Carbohydrates: 4g; Fiber: 0g; Sugar: 2g; Protein: 20g

Swiss Chard and Smoked Salmon Cups

Dairy-Free, Gluten-Free, No Added Sugar, Omega-3-Rich, Soy-Free
Prep time: 10 minutes / **Cook time:** 10 minutes • **Makes 12 muffin cups**

I'm a big fan of versatile recipes to cut down on food waste and expense, and this one is no different. Replace the parsley with fresh dill, add cream cheese or nutritional yeast, substitute any onion for the chives, or change the greens.

1 tablespoon extra-virgin olive oil

4 large Swiss chard leaves, ribs removed and chopped

4 ounces smoked salmon, coarsely chopped

10 large eggs (pastured or omega-3 labeled)

1 tablespoon water

1 scallion, white and green parts, minced

2 tablespoons chopped fresh parsley

½ teaspoon freshly ground black pepper

1 teaspoon Dijon mustard (optional)

Freshly squeezed lemon juice, for serving (optional)

1. Preheat the oven to 350°F. Lightly grease a 12-cup muffin pan with oil (or use silicone or parchment baking cups). Equally divide the Swiss chard and salmon among all muffin cups.

2. In a medium bowl, combine the eggs, water, scallions, parsley, pepper, and mustard (if using). Whisk, then pour the egg mixture into each muffin cup, filling nearly to the top.

3. Bake for 22 minutes, then let cool for 5 minutes. Squeeze fresh lemon juice on top (if using), and serve.

VARIATION TIP: For a non-seafood option, replace the smoked salmon with diced ham, though this will drop the omega-3 content substantially. Also, for dairy eaters, you can add ½ cup of shredded cheese (when using ham) for a more complex flavor.

Per Serving (2 muffins): Calories: 169; Total fat: 11g; Saturated fat: 3g; Sodium: 566mg; Carbohydrates: 2g; Fiber: 1g; Sugar: 1g; Protein: 15g

Chocolate Protein Cauliflower Smoothie

Dairy-Free, Gluten-Free, No Added Sugar, Nut-free, Soy-Free, Vegetarian
Prep time: 5 minutes · **Serves** 1

High-sugar, low-fiber smoothies won't keep you satisfied for very long and can spike blood sugars, requiring more insulin from the pancreas. A blood sugar drop then follows and can predispose you to mindless snacking. Repeat this process consistently, and you may find yourself perpetuating inflammation rather than alleviating it. This smoothie comes to the rescue with protein, vegetables, and healthy fat. I love chocolate, so starting my day with this nutrient-packed smoothie just feels right.

1½ cups unsweetened vanilla plant-based milk (I use a flax-based milk)
1 serving chocolate protein powder
½ cup frozen cauliflower
2 prunes
1 cup fresh baby spinach

6 ice cubes
1 tablespoon almond butter or ¼ avocado (optional)
1 tablespoon ground flaxseed or chia seeds (optional)
Water, to thin, as needed

In a blender, combine the plant-based milk, protein powder, cauliflower, prunes, spinach, ice, almond butter (if using), and flaxseed (if using). Blend until smooth. Add water as needed to thin and blend sufficiently.

VARIATION TIP: For a mocha chocolate smoothie, substitute black coffee for 4 ounces of the plant milk. For a vegan option, make sure to use chocolate pea protein or your preferred vegetarian protein choice.

Per Serving: Calories: 271; Total fat: 4g; Saturated fat: 0g; Sodium: 330mg; Carbohydrates: 27g; Fiber: 6g; Sugar: 13g; Protein: 29g

Triple Berry Granola Cups

Dairy-Free, Gluten-Free, No Added Sugar (option), Soy-Free, Vegetarian
Prep time: 5 minutes / **Cook time:** 25 minutes • **Makes 12 muffin cups**

Need a hearty and make-ahead breakfast for busy mornings? These granola cups avoid the pitfalls of traditional sugary breakfasts and don't contain any added sugars (or banana), yet taste surprisingly sweet and complex. Crunchy granola on top, warm berry oatmeal on the bottom, and filled with fiber, omega-3s, and prebiotics, these are sure to be a new household favorite. My family loves to top them with almond butter.

Extra-virgin olive oil, for greasing
1½ cups rolled oats
¼ cup ground flaxseed
1½ tablespoons cinnamon
¼ teaspoon salt
1 cup unsweetened vanilla almond
  milk yogurt

⅓ cup water
1½ cups frozen mixed berries (such as
  blueberries, blackberries, and raspberries)
Honey or maple syrup (optional)

1. Preheat the oven to 400°F. Lightly grease a muffin pan with oil (or use silicone baking cups).

2. In a medium bowl, combine the oats, flaxseed, cinnamon, and salt. Add the yogurt and water and stir to combine. Gently fold in the frozen mixed berries.

3. Spoon the batter into the muffin cups, filling them nearly full. Bake for 25 minutes or until golden on the top. Let the muffins cool for 5 minutes, plate, drizzle honey or maple syrup (if using) on top, and serve.

VARIATION TIP: To boost the omega-3 content of this recipe, fold in ¼ cup of finely chopped walnuts along with the berries.

Per Serving (2 muffins): Calories: 184; Total fat: 5g; Saturated fat: 1g; Sodium: 126mg; Carbohydrates: 30g; Fiber: 7g; Sugar: 7g; Protein: 8g

Vibrant Green Smoothie

Dairy-Free, Gluten-Free, No Added Sugar, Soy-Free, Vegan
Prep time: 5 minutes • **Serves** 2

Smoothies are a quick way to pack in anti-inflammatory ingredients, and this version is loaded with nutritious spinach and ginger, as well as healthy fats from the avocado to improve absorption of vitamins, minerals, and antioxidants. Adding some fruit but no juice helps add a touch of sweetness without the sugar overload. While not required, adding cilantro adds another layer of fresh flavor, plus anti-inflammatory quercetin and more antioxidants, to the smoothie.

3 cups baby spinach

Juice of 1 lemon

½ avocado

2 Granny Smith apples, cored and chopped

¼ cup cilantro leaves (optional)

1-inch piece ginger, peeled

2 cups water

1 cup crushed ice

In a blender, combine the spinach, lemon juice, avocado, apple, cilantro (if using), ginger, water, and ice. Blend until smooth.

VARIATION TIP: I like to substitute either fresh-brewed or leftover green tea for the water for an extra antioxidant and anti-inflammatory kick.

Per Serving: Calories: 199; Total fat: 8g; Saturated fat: 0g; Sodium: 42mg; Carbohydrates: 30g; Fiber: 9g; Sugar: 21g; Protein: 3g

Quick Greens and Cauliflower Bowl

Dairy-Free, Gluten-Free, No Added Sugar, Nut-Free, Soy-Free, Vegan, Vegetarian
Prep time: 5 minutes / **Cook time:** 5 minutes • **Serves 1**

Cruciferous vegetables in the morning? Well, why not? These hot, tender-crisp vegetables make for a light, nourishing breakfast that's ready in minutes. If you'd like extra protein, toss in a handful of beans or flake in a few chunks of left-over salmon.

4 kale leaves, thoroughly washed
  and chopped
1½ cups cauliflower florets
½ avocado, chopped

2 teaspoons freshly squeezed lemon juice,
  or more to taste
1 teaspoon extra-virgin olive oil
Pinch salt
Pinch pepper

1. Fill a medium saucepan with 2 inches of water and insert a steamer basket. Bring to a boil over high heat.

2. Put the kale and cauliflower in the basket. Cover and steam for 5 minutes.

3. Transfer the vegetables to a medium bowl. Toss with the avocado, lemon juice, olive oil, salt, and pepper.

PREP TIP: Chop the cauliflower and kale the night before, put them in the steamer basket, and refrigerate them overnight. In the morning, they'll be ready to cook when you are. Alternatively, choose prewashed, pre-chopped packages of kale and cauliflower to further minimize your prep time.

Per Serving: Calories: Calories: 317; Total fat: 21g; Saturated fat: 2g; Sodium: 258mg; Carbohydrates: 29g; Fiber: 15g; Sugar: 7g; Protein: 11g

Stovetop Steel-Cut Oats with Banana, Cherries, and Almonds

Dairy-Free, Gluten-Free, No Added Sugar, Soy-Free, Vegan
Prep time: 5 minutes / **Cook time:** 15 minutes • **Serves 6**

You can whip up these hearty oats on the stove in less than 30 minutes. Naturally sweetened with banana, these steel-cut oats are full of fiber and are complemented by delicious anti-inflammatory cherries and almonds. To save time, cook the oats ahead, and you can have this recipe done in barely 5 minutes.

2 cups steel-cut oats
4½ cups unsweetened dairy-free milk
1 spotted large banana, fresh or frozen and
   thawed, sliced

2 cups tart cherries, fresh or frozen, halved
   and pitted
½ cup slivered almonds, chopped
1 tablespoon cinnamon (optional)

1. In a large saucepan, combine the oats and milk and bring to a boil over medium-high heat. Reduce the heat to medium-low and simmer for 15 minutes, or until the oats are soft.

2. Remove from the heat and add the banana. Cover the saucepan for 2 to 3 minutes to soften the banana. Mash or stir the softened banana into the oats until incorporated. Add the cherries and almonds, mixing to combine.

3. Serve immediately, garnished with cinnamon (if using) and more cherries or almonds, if desired.

STORAGE: Refrigerate for up to 4 days. To serve, add 1 to 2 tablespoons of milk to the oats to thin them slightly and microwave for 1 to 2 minutes, until heated through.

VARIATION TIP: Use rolled oats instead of steel-cut oats for a softer, more traditional oatmeal texture. To do this, reduce the cooking time to 10 minutes. Mix in ¼ cup raisins with the banana for a sweeter flavor or add an extra ½ banana.

Per Serving: Calories: 288; Total fat: 9g; Saturated fat: 1g; Sodium: 100mg; Carbohydrates: 45g; Fiber: 8g; Sugar: 9g; Protein: 10g

Chia Breakfast Pudding Your Way

Dairy-Free, Gluten-Free, No Added Sugar (option), Soy-Free
Prep time: 5 minutes • **Serves 4**

This chia pudding is rich in calcium, protein, and anti-inflammatory omega-3 fats, and you can create endless variations. Start with the basic recipe and play around with the liquid, sweeteners, and other add-ins. You can even create a topping "buffet" so everyone can customize their own bowl. For a protein powder, I like to use a stevia-sweetened or unsweetened option, such as Vital Proteins unflavored or vanilla collagen peptides, to minimize added sugars.

¾ cup chia seeds

½ cup hemp seeds

2¼ cups unsweetened vanilla almond or other plant-based milk (not canned)

½ cup unsweetened dried cherries or raisins

4 scoops dairy-free vanilla protein powder

Optional ingredient swaps or add-ins:

Dairy-free milk (almond milk, cashew milk, flax milk, hemp milk, oat milk)

Dried fruit (raisins, blueberries, apricots, dates, goji berries, apples)

Grains (use ¼ cup of buckwheat groats instead of the chia seeds)

Sweeteners (maple syrup, raw honey, stevia, allulose, or coconut sugar)

Make it fancy (vanilla, cinnamon, dairy-free chocolate chips or cacao nibs, walnuts, pumpkin seeds, ground ginger)

Fresh fruit (berries, peaches or pears)

1. In a medium bowl, stir together the chia seeds, hemp seeds, coconut milk, and cherries, ensuring that the chia is completely mixed with the milk. Whisk in the protein powder until all clumps are incorporated.

2. Cover the bowl and refrigerate overnight. In the morning, stir and serve.

PREP TIP: If you don't like the consistency of whole chia seeds, blend them with the milk before adding the remaining ingredients. This will produce a smoother pudding and distribute the sweetness more evenly.

Per Serving (¾ cup, no add-ins): Calories: 441; Total fat: 24g; Saturated fat: 2g; Sodium: 151mg; Carbohydrates: 38g; Fiber: 17g; Sugar: 12g; Protein: 24g

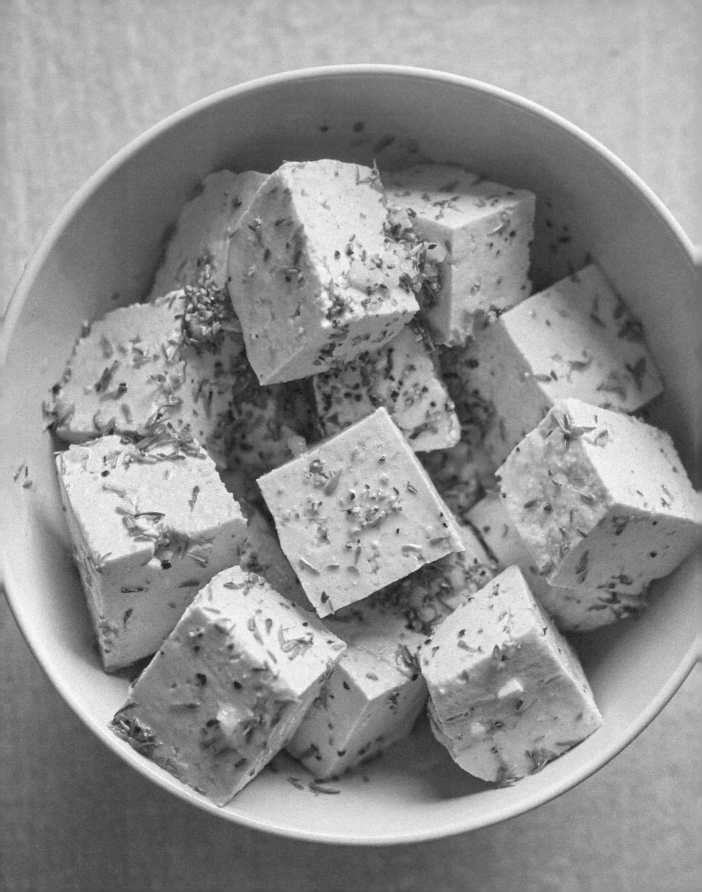

CHAPTER 3

SNACKS AND APPETIZERS

Chilled Smoked Salmon and Cauliflower Dip

Gluten-Free, No Added Sugar, Nut-free, Soy-Free

Prep time: 5 minutes, plus 30 minutes to chill • **Serves** 8

This powerhouse dip is inspired by two flavors I'm fond of—lox bagels and Buffalo sauce. Why not marry the two into a healthy dip? The yogurt imparts probiotics and a creamy texture, while the smoked salmon and cauliflower ramp up the anti-inflammatory nutrition. Dill is a complementary flavor for salmon, so it's an ideal pairing, but you can also substitute a dill spice blend or a no-sodium garden vegetable blend.

1 cup nonfat Greek yogurt

2 ounces smoked salmon, chopped

2 tablespoons Buffalo sauce (I recommend Frank's RedHot Original Buffalo Sauce)

½ cup steamer bag cauliflower rice (fresh or frozen), cooked and cooled

1 teaspoon fresh or dried dill

Carrot sticks, celery sticks, or seed crackers to dip (optional)

In a small bowl, combine the yogurt, salmon, Buffalo sauce, cooled cauliflower rice, and dill. Chill for at least 30 minutes. Serve with vegetable or crackers of choice, if using.

VARIATION TIP: For dairy-free eaters, replace the Greek yogurt with ¾ cup cashew cream cheese and ¼ cup dairy-free ranch dressing. I love the Tessamae brand.

Per Serving (2 tablespoons): Calories: 28; Total fat: 1g; Saturated fat: 0g; Sodium: 177mg; Carbohydrates: 2g; Fiber: 0g; Sugar: 1g; Protein: 4g

Easy Beet Salsa

Dairy-Free, Gluten-Free, No Added Sugar, Nut-free, Soy-Free, Vegan
Prep time: 5 minutes, plus 30 minutes to chill / **Cook time:** 30 minutes • **Serves** 6

Traditional tomato salsa is easy to come by at grocery stores and restaurants, but this unique and nutrient-dense salsa will wow you and give your body an anti-inflammatory boost. Beets are rich in nitrates and betalains, both powerful compounds to help filter the bloodstream and reduce inflammation. I like to serve this with carrot sticks, bean tortilla chips, plantain chips, and as a topper for salads.

2 large red beets (no greens)
½ medium white onion
1 bunch cilantro, stems discarded
1 jalapeño pepper (seeded for less heat)

Juice of 2 limes
¼ teaspoon salt
1-inch piece ginger, peeled (optional)

1. Fill a medium saucepan with 1 to 2 inches of water. Insert a steamer basket, put the beets inside, cover, and bring to a boil over high heat.

2. Reduce the heat to low and steam for about 30 minutes. When the beets are cool enough to handle, rub off the peels, then quarter the beets.

3. In the bowl of a food processor, combine the beets, onion, cilantro, jalapeño, lime juice, salt, and ginger (if using). Pulse until well combined and minced. Add more lime juice or water, 1 tablespoon at a time, as needed to thin to desired consistency. Taste and season with more salt, if desired.

4. Chill for at least 30 minutes before serving. Store in the refrigerator for up to 3 days.

VARIATION TIP: If you prefer a more traditional salsa, but want to still enjoy the benefits of beets, add 1 medium tomato after step 2.

Per Serving (¼ cup): Calories: 20; Total fat: 0g; Saturated fat: 0g; Sodium: 119mg; Carbohydrates: 5g; Fiber: 1g; Sugar: 3g; Protein: 0g

Halibut Ceviche

Dairy-Free, Gluten-Free, No Added Sugar, Omega-3-Rich, Nut-Free, Soy-Free

Prep time: 10 minutes, plus 1 hour to chill / **Cook time:** 1 hour • **Serves 4**

Ceviche, a South American favorite, is one of the few ways to enjoy fish without cooking it. It's often served on warm days. Halibut is a wonderful omega-3-rich fish for those who prefer to avoid "fishy" fish. When halibut is out of season or too expensive for the budget, barramundi is a great substitute.

8 ounces frozen, thawed halibut, patted dry
  with paper towels and diced
1 medium tomato, diced
½ small white onion, diced
½ bunch cilantro, stems discarded, diced

Juice of 3 limes, about ⅓ cup
½ teaspoon salt
Chips to dip, or tortillas or lettuce for wraps
  (optional)

1. In a medium glass dish, combine the halibut, tomato, onion, cilantro, lime juice, and salt and stir well.

2. Chill for at least 1 hour or until the fish is opaque and "cooked" by the lime juice. Serve with chips, on tortillas, or in lettuce wraps (if desired).

VARIATION TIP: Flavor combination possibilities are endless with ceviche. Add mango for sweetness, avocado for richness, and/or serrano peppers for more heat.

Per Serving (½ cup): Calories: 69; Total fat: 1g; Saturated fat: 0g; Sodium:332mg; Carbohydrates: 5g; Fiber: 1g; Sugar: 2g; Protein: 11g

Turmeric Sauerkraut Deviled Eggs

Gluten-Free, No Added Sugar, Nut-free, Omega-3 Rich, Soy-Free, Vegetarian
Prep time: 10 minutes, plus 30 minutes to chill / **Cook time:** 15 minutes
Makes 24 deviled eggs

These aren't your ordinary deviled eggs. Mayonnaise is replaced with probiotic-rich yogurt, and relish with probiotic-rich sauerkraut. Choose pastured or omega-3-rich eggs, and you are well on your way to anti-inflammatory snacking.

1 dozen large eggs

½ cup plain nonfat Greek yogurt

2 tablespoons raw sauerkraut, minced, plus
   1 tablespoon juice

1 tablespoon prepared mustard

½ teaspoon ground turmeric

½ teaspoon freshly ground black pepper

¼ teaspoon salt

Paprika, for garnish (optional)

1. Fill a large saucepan with water and add the eggs. Bring the water and eggs to a rolling boil, then remove from the heat and cover for 14 minutes.

2. Remove the eggs and cool in an ice bath for 5 minutes. Peel the eggs and halve them lengthwise. Carefully scoop out the yolks—leaving the whites intact—and transfer the yolks to a medium bowl.

3. Mash the yolks with a fork and stir in the yogurt, sauerkraut, juice, mustard, turmeric, pepper, and salt.

4. Scoop the yolk filling into the empty egg whites, and sprinkle with paprika, if desired. Chill for at least 30 minutes before serving.

PREP TIP: Farm-fresh eggs (which have tightly bound membranes) need to be cooked differently from store-bought eggs. First, bring the water to a low boil, then carefully slip the eggs into the boiling water. Lower the heat, simmer for 8 minutes, then proceed to step 2.

Per Serving (2 halves): Calories: 73; Total fat: 5g; Saturated fat: 2g; Sodium: 144mg; Carbohydrates: 1g; Fiber: 0g; Sugar: 0g; Protein: 6g

Savory Lentil Flatbread

Dairy-Free, Gluten-Free, No Added Sugar, Soy-Free, Vegan
Prep time: 5 minutes, plus 3 hours to soak / **Cook time:** 25 minutes • **Serves** 6

Dosa is a South Indian staple and a healthy, high-protein, and high-fiber alternative to traditional breads. For more Indian-inspired flavor, substitute ¼ teaspoon of fenugreek seeds for the scallion and garlic.

1 cup dry red lentils

3 cups water, divided

1 teaspoon sea salt

½ teaspoon garlic powder

2 scallions, green and white parts, minced

2 tablespoons minced fresh cilantro

Olive oil, for cooking

Cilantro chutney, for serving (optional)

1. In a medium bowl, stir together the lentils and 1½ cups of water. Let soak for 3 hours or up to overnight on the counter.

2. Rinse and drain the lentils and pour them into a blender. Add the remaining 1½ cups of water, the salt, and the garlic powder and blend until creamy. Stir in the scallion and cilantro. Add water, 1 tablespoon at a time, until you reach a thin pancake batter consistency.

3. Place a large nonstick skillet on medium-low heat. Brush the skillet with olive oil. Add a ¼-cup scoop of batter to the skillet and flatten into a pancake, about 4 to 6 inches in diameter, with the back of the scoop

4. Cook for 2 to 3 minutes, flip, then cook for another 2 to 3 minutes. When the flatbread is cooked and ready to be flipped, it will loosen from the pan. Be careful to flip before it burns. Transfer the flatbread to a rack to cool. Repeat with the remaining batter.

5. Dip in cilantro chutney, if desired, or serve alongside curries or soup.

PREP TIP: Refrigerate the batter for up to 2 days. Once cooked, these can be refrigerated for up to 5 days or frozen for up to 3 months. Reheat in a toaster oven or in a dry, warm pan.

Per Serving (1 flatbread): Calories: 124; Total fat: 1g; Saturated fat: 0g; Sodium: 431mg; Carbohydrates: 21g; Fiber: 4g; Sugar: 0g; Protein: 8g

Roasted Butternut Squash Mash

Dairy-Free, Gluten-Free, No Added Sugar, Soy-Free, Vegan
Prep time: 10 minutes / **Cook time:** 30 minutes • **Serves 4**

To mash or not to mash? They're irresistible mashed, but you can also enjoy these roasted vegetables as is or as part of a salad. Either way, carrots and apples add a nice sweetness to this comfort food. The carotenoids in the squash and carrots help reduce inflammation and cardiovascular disease risk, well worth switching it up from regular mashed potatoes.

3 cups cubed butternut squash

1 cup coarsely chopped carrot

1 large green apple, peeled, cored, and chopped

3 tablespoons extra-virgin olive oil

1 teaspoon salt

¼ teaspoon freshly ground black pepper

½ cup unsweetened almond milk

1 teaspoon of minced fresh herbs (such as sage or rosemary)

1. Preheat the oven to 375°F.

2. Combine the squash, carrot, and apple in a large bowl. Add the oil, salt, and pepper and toss to mix well.

3. Transfer the vegetables to a parchment-paper-lined baking sheet and roast until the vegetables are tender and lightly browned, 20 to 30 minutes.

4. Return the vegetables to the bowl.

5. Using a potato masher, mash the vegetables, add the milk, and stir until mostly smooth, with a few lumps. Sprinkle the herbs on top. Serve immediately.

VARIATION TIP: For a twist, try this recipe using sweet potatoes instead of butternut squash.

PREP TIP: Look in the produce section for baby carrots and pre-cubed butternut squash to minimize your prep time.

Per Serving: Calories: 191; Total fat: 11g; Saturated fat: 1g; Sodium: 432mg; Carbohydrates: 22g; Fiber: 4g; Sugar: 9g; Protein: 1g

Garlic-Herb Marinated Tempeh or Tofu

Dairy-Free, Gluten-Free, No Added Sugar, Nut-Free, Vegan
Prep time: 10 minutes, plus 20 minutes to marinate / **Cook time:** 20 minutes • **Serves** 3

Tempeh and tofu have very subtle flavors on their own, but they can be dressed up easily. Marinating these plant-based proteins in a savory broth, tangy vinegar, and anti-inflammatory herbs and spices makes a wonderful base for many dishes.

8 ounces tempeh or 14 ounces
   extra-firm tofu
2 tablespoons olive oil
¼ cup vegetable broth or water
1 tablespoon white wine vinegar

3 garlic cloves, minced
1½ teaspoons dried thyme
½ teaspoon salt
½ teaspoon freshly ground black pepper

1. Preheat the oven to 400°F. Line a baking sheet with parchment paper.

2. If using tempeh, slice it crosswise into 1-inch-thick slices. If using tofu, press the tops and sides gently with a paper towel to remove extra water. Halve it lengthwise and press the slices again with a paper towel. Cut the tofu into 1-inch cubes.

3. In a large bowl, combine the oil, broth, vinegar, garlic, thyme, salt, and pepper. Put the tempeh or tofu in the marinade and use a spoon to coat it thoroughly. Let it marinate for at least 10 minutes, then flip or toss and marinate for 10 minutes more.

4. Pour the tofu or tempeh and marinade onto the sheet pan in a single layer and bake for 15 to 20 minutes, until the tempeh or tofu is slightly browned.

STORAGE: Refrigerate in a sealed container for up to 6 days. To reheat, microwave for 1 minute.

Per Serving: Calories: 233; Total fat: 17g; Saturated fat: 3g; Sodium: 396mg; Carbohydrates: 9g; Fiber: 0g; Sugar: 0g; Protein: 14g

Garlic-Lime Black Beans

Dairy-Free, Gluten-Free, No Added Sugar, Nut-Free, Soy-Free, Vegan
Prep time: 5 minutes / **Cook time:** 10 minutes • **Serves 5**

A side of black beans doesn't have to be boring. This recipe is a flavor-packed and versatile staple that goes with so many other dishes in this book. You can whip it up in minutes, using canned beans to save time. Like to meal-prep meals for the week? These beans are the perfect easy and filling side to make ahead.

1 tablespoon olive oil

2 garlic cloves, minced

2 (15.5-ounce) cans black beans, drained and rinsed

Juice of 1 to 2 limes

1 teaspoon ground cumin

½ teaspoon salt

1. In a medium saucepan, heat the oil over medium heat. Add the garlic and sauté for 1 to 3 minutes until it starts turning golden brown.

2. Add the black beans, lime juice, cumin, and salt and stir occasionally for 4 to 6 minutes more, mashing some of the beans to create a varied texture. Cool before storing.

STORAGE: Store in the refrigerator for up to 5 days. To serve, microwave for 2 minutes until heated through or quickly warm in a small saucepan on the stovetop.

VARIATION TIP: Play with spice levels to taste. Try adding another clove of garlic or adjusting the level of cumin. To give the beans a kick of heat, try adding freshly ground black pepper, chili powder, or chipotle chili powder.

Per Serving: Calories: 165; Total fat: 3g; Saturated fat: 0g; Sodium: 235mg; Carbohydrates: 26g; Fiber: 9g; Sugar: 0g; Protein: 9g

Kale Chips

Dairy-Free, Gluten-Free, Nut-Free, No Added Sugar, Soy-Free, Vegan
Prep time: 15 minutes / **Cook time:** 20 minutes • **Serves** 4

Even though kale chips are readily available at the grocery store, they can be expensive. This recipe makes delicious chips at a fraction of the price. Better yet, when you make your own, you know what's in them and are assured you're getting maximum nutrition. If you like it spicy, add a pinch of red pepper flakes to the kale before baking. Enjoy within 24 hours because they lose their crunch quickly.

1 large bunch kale, washed and thoroughly dried, stems removed, leaves cut into 2-inch pieces
2 tablespoons extra-virgin olive oil

Juice of ½ lemon
1 teaspoon sea salt
1 tablespoon nutritional yeast

1. Preheat the oven to 275°F. Line a baking sheet with parchment paper.

2. In a large bowl, use your hands to mix the kale, olive oil, and lemon until the kale is evenly coated.

3. Transfer the kale to the baking sheet and sprinkle with sea salt and nutritional yeast.

4. Bake, turning the kale leaves halfway through, until crispy, about 20 minutes.

PREP TIP: Cut down on prep time by using 4 cups of prewashed, pre-chopped kale.

Per Serving: Calories: 72; Total fat: 7g; Saturated fat: 1g; Sodium: 388mg; Carbohydrates: 2g; Fiber: 1g; Sugar: 1g; Protein: 1g

Lima Bean Hummus

Dairy-Free, Gluten-Free, No Added Sugar, Nut-Free, Soy-Free, Vegan
Prep time: 10 minutes / **Cook time:** 10 minutes • **Serves** 10

This hummus tastes great on seed crackers, chips, and with fresh vegetables, such as carrots, bell peppers, cucumber, broccoli, cauliflower, and celery. This recipe uses frozen lima beans, but you can easily replace them with canned or cooked chickpeas or replace half with green peas.

2 cups frozen lima beans

⅓ cup tahini

Juice of 2 large lemons, plus more to taste

2 garlic cloves, halved

¾ teaspoon salt

1 teaspoon ground cumin

2 to 4 tablespoons water

3 tablespoons olive oil

¼ cup chopped parsley (optional)

1. Cook the frozen lima beans as per package instructions. Maximum cook time is typically 8 to 10 minutes in the microwave or longer on the stove.

2. In a food processor or blender, combine the lima beans, tahini, lemon juice, garlic, salt, cumin, and 2 tablespoons of water. Puree the mixture until it's smooth. If it needs more liquid, add up to 2 more tablespoons of water, 1 tablespoon at a time. With the food processor running, slowly drizzle in the olive oil 1 tablespoon at a time, blending well to incorporate after each addition.

3. Taste and season with more salt or lemon as desired. Stir in the parsley (if using) and serve.

STORAGE: Refrigerate for up to 7 days or freeze for up to 3 months. If frozen, thaw in the refrigerator overnight before serving.

PREP TIP: A food processor is best for this recipe, so you can drizzle the olive oil in slowly while the motor is running. If you're using a blender, add 1 tablespoon of oil at a time and pulse 5 to 10 times to incorporate.

Per Serving: Calories: 130; Total fat: 9g; Saturated fat: 1g; Sodium: 201mg; Carbohydrates: 11g; Fiber: 3g; Sugar: 0g; Protein: 4g

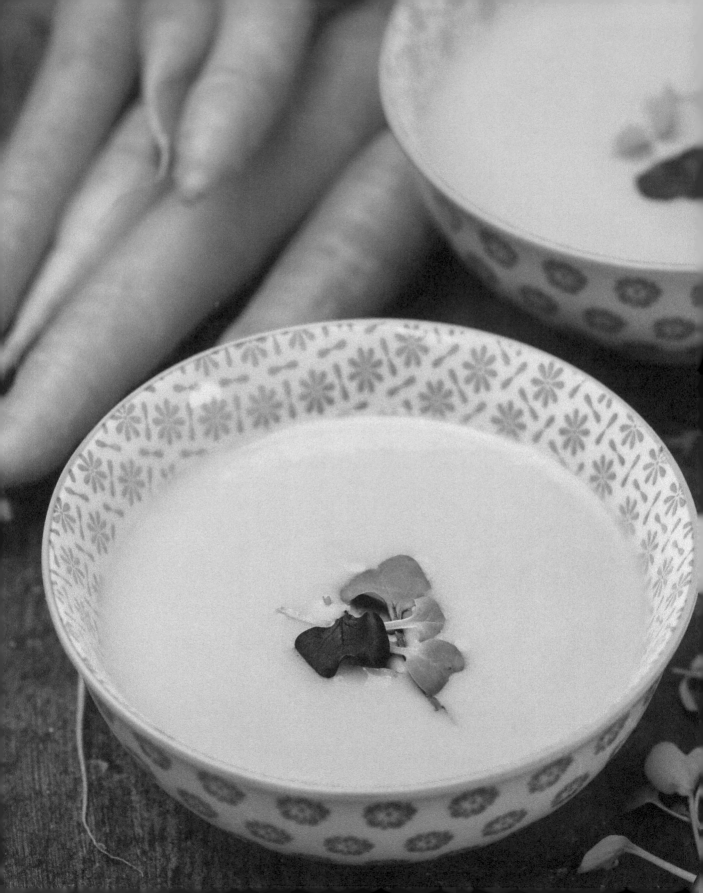

CHAPTER 4

SOUPS AND SALADS

Rotisserie Chicken, Kale, and White Bean Soup

Dairy-Free, Gluten-Free, No Added Sugar, Soy-Free
Prep time: 5 minutes / **Cook time:** 1 hour • **Serves 4**

According to the Harvard School of Public Health, kale is one of the most nutrient-dense vegetables available. This recipe combines the powerhouse ingredients of kale and bone broth for phytochemicals and healing collagen. Using precooked chicken along with apple cider vinegar speeds up the collagen extracting process from the chicken bones. However, if you have the time, you can simmer the bones for up to six hours to extract the most collagen. Although this soup doesn't require lemon, adding it provides a brightness and acidity that makes this soup smell and taste glorious.

1 rotisserie chicken

1 tablespoon apple cider vinegar

2 tablespoons extra-virgin olive oil

1 bunch scallions, green and white parts, sliced, divided

1 bunch fresh kale, ribs removed, chopped (or substitute 12 ounces frozen chopped kale)

2 (15-ounce) cans cannellini beans, drained and rinsed (optional)

2 tablespoons Italian herb seasoning

1 teaspoon salt

1 teaspoon freshly ground black pepper

1 lemon, quartered (optional)

1. Separate the meat from the bones on the rotisserie chicken. Put the meat in a bowl, gently pull it apart into bite-size pieces, and set it aside.

2. In a large pot, combine the chicken carcass/bones, enough water to cover, and the apple cider vinegar. Bring to a boil over medium-high heat, reduce the heat to low, and simmer uncovered for at least 1 hour. Strain the stock through a fine-mesh sieve—discarding the solids—and set aside.

3. Heat the oil in a medium saucepan on medium-high heat. Sauté the scallions for 2 to 3 minutes until softened. Add the kale and sauté until softened and wilted, 2 to 3 minutes. Add half of the chicken meat (reserving the rest for another use), beans (if using), 5 cups stock, Italian seasoning, salt, and pepper.

4. Cook for 15 minutes to soften the beans and reduce the liquid. Add more stock as needed to maintain desired liquid volume. Refrigerate remaining stock if desired.

5. Taste, and season with more salt and pepper as needed. If using, add the juice of a quarter of lemon (or more) to each bowl before serving.

VARIATION TIP: Replace the kale with spinach. Both are in the cruciferous family. Any white canned bean will work; don't worry if you don't have cannellini on hand. White navy bean, Great Northern beans, and even chickpeas are great, though each bean will provide a different texture to the soup (Great Northern beans are the softest).

Per Serving (2 cups): Calories: 365; Total fat: 9g; Saturated fat: 1g; Sodium: 531mg; Carbohydrates: 36g; Fiber: 15g; Sugar: 2g; Protein: 37g

Chipotle Sweet Potato and Cauliflower Soup

Dairy-Free, Gluten-Free, No Added Sugar, Soy-Free, Vegan
Prep time: 10 minutes / **Cook time:** 20 minutes • **Serves 4**

Abundant research has confirmed the anti-inflammatory benefits of both carotenoids—found in sweet potatoes and other red, yellow, or orange vegetables—and sulfur compounds in cauliflower and other cruciferous vegetables. This soup combines both powerhouse ingredients along with smoky spice from the chipotle peppers and acidity from the lime juice to create a tasty, healthy, warming soup. Serve this alongside Savory Lentil Flatbread (page 38) or Walnut Bean Burgers (page 61).

2 tablespoons extra-virgin olive oil

1 onion, chopped

2 cups cauliflower rice, fresh or frozen

2 medium sweet potatoes, peeled, washed, and chopped

2 chipotle peppers in adobo, from 1 (7½-ounce) can, chopped

5 cups water, or vegetable broth

1 teaspoon salt

1 teaspoon freshly ground black pepper

1 teaspoon ground cumin (optional)

Juice of 2 limes

1. Heat the oil in a large saucepan over medium heat and sauté the onion for 3 to 4 minutes until caramelized. Add the cauliflower rice and sauté 2 to 3 minutes.

2. Add the sweet potatoes, chipotle peppers, 1 tablespoon of sauce from the can, water, salt, black pepper, and cumin (if using).

3. Bring to a boil, reduce the heat to low, and simmer for 20 minutes to cook the sweet potato and reduce the liquid.

4. Remove the soup from the heat and puree using an immersion blender or transfer the soup to a blender and carefully blend (it will be hot). Transfer it back to the saucepan and stir in the lime juice. If desired, add more water or broth, ½ cup at a time, until you reach your preferred consistency.

5. Taste, season with more salt and black pepper as desired, and serve.

PREP TIP: Replace the cauliflower rice with half a head of cauliflower, stem removed. Leftover cooked sweet potato works, too, and will allow a faster cook time to finish the soup.

Per Serving: Calories: 147; Total fat: 7g; Saturated fat: 1g; Sodium: 625mg; Carbohydrates: 21g; Fiber: 4g; Sugar: 6g; Protein: 3g

Carrot-Ginger Soup

Dairy-Free, Gluten-Free, No Added Sugar, Soy-Free, Vegan
Prep time: 10 minutes / **Cook time:** 30 minutes • **Serves 6**

This creamy soup combines two powerful anti-inflammatory ingredients in one comforting bowl. Depending on your tolerance for ginger, add more or less than what is called for here. This is a family staple for us, especially in the winter months.

1 large onion, peeled and coarsely chopped

4¼ cups plus 3 tablespoons water, divided

8 carrots, peeled and coarsely chopped
(see Tip)

1½-inch piece fresh ginger, sliced thin
(see Tip)

1½ teaspoons salt

2 cups canned coconut milk

¼ cup whole almonds

1 to 2 limes, quartered, for serving
(optional)

Microgreens, for garnishing (optional)

1. In a large stockpot over medium heat, sauté the onion in 3 tablespoons of water for about 5 minutes, or until soft.

2. Add the carrots, the remaining 4¼ cups of water, the ginger, and the salt. Bring to a boil. Reduce the heat to low, cover, and simmer for 20 minutes.

3. Add the coconut milk and let it heat for 4 to 5 minutes.

4. In a blender, combine the almonds and the soup and blend until creamy, working in batches if necessary and taking care with the hot liquid.

5. Squeeze a quarter or two of lime into each bowl or garnish with microgreens before serving, if desired.

PREP TIP: You don't have to peel the carrots or ginger if they're organic—leave the skin on and wash them well.

Per Serving (1½ cups): Calories: 228; Total fat: 19g; Saturated fat: 14g; Sodium: 642mg; Carbohydrates: 15g; Fiber: 4g; Sugar: 6g; Protein: 4g

Whitefish Chowder

Dairy-Free, Gluten-Free, No Added Sugar, Omega-3-Rich, Soy-Free
Prep time: 10 minutes / **Cook time:** 35 minutes • **Serves 6**

Coconut milk lends this minimalist chowder its delicious creaminess. Use the full-fat variety, as it will add a satisfying thickness to the bowl. If you have any extra anti-inflammatory or aromatic vegetables such as onion, garlic, or celery kicking around your kitchen, throw them in, too.

4 carrots, peeled and cut into ½-inch pieces

3 sweet potatoes, peeled and cut into
   ½-inch pieces

3 cups full-fat coconut milk

2 cups water

1 teaspoon celery seed or ground thyme
   (optional)

1 teaspoon salt

1 teaspoon freshly ground black pepper

10½ ounces whitefish, skinless and firm,
   such as barramundi, cut into chunks

Grated zest of 1 lime

Juice of 3 limes

¼ cup minced parsley (optional)

1. In a large stockpot, combine the carrots, sweet potatoes, coconut milk, water, celery seed (if using), salt, and pepper. Bring to a boil over high heat, reduce the heat to low, cover, and simmer for 20 minutes.

2. Transfer half of the soup to a blender and puree. Return the puree to the stockpot. Add the fish chunks.

3. Cook for 12 to 15 minutes more, or until the fish is tender and hot. Add the lime zest and juice and stir. Garnish with fresh parsley (if using) and serve hot.

VARIATION TIP: If you don't like the taste of coconut milk or need to keep your saturated fat low, substitute almond milk. To achieve the same creamy texture, blend three-fourths of the soup before returning it to the pot.

Per Serving (1⅔ cup): Calories: 336; Total fat: 24g; Saturated fat: 21g; Sodium: 589mg; Carbohydrates: 22g; Fiber: 5g; Sugar: 5g; Protein: 11g

Homestyle Red Lentil Stew

Dairy-Free, Gluten-Free, No Added Sugar, Soy-Free, Vegan
Prep time: 10 minutes / **Cook time:** 35 minutes • **Serves 6**

Like all lentils, the red variety is packed with protein, fiber, B vitamins, and energy-boosting iron. What differentiates red lentils from its siblings, other than its bright red-orange color, is the super-quick cooking time. Red lentils are so little they disintegrate as they cook, yielding a thick, stick-to-your-ribs texture that doesn't need blending. Hooray for one less step!

2 tablespoons extra-virgin olive oil

2 onions, peeled and finely diced

4 celery stalks, finely diced

6½ cups water

3 cups red lentils

2 zucchini, finely diced

1 teaspoon dried oregano

1 teaspoon salt, plus more as needed

1 teaspoon freshly ground black pepper, plus more as needed

1. In a large stockpot set over medium heat, add the oil and sauté the onions and celery for about 5 minutes, until soft.

2. Add the water, lentils, zucchini, oregano, salt, and pepper. Bring to a boil, reduce the heat to low, cover, and simmer for 30 minutes, stirring occasionally, until the lentils are soft.

3. Taste, and adjust the seasoning if necessary.

VARIATION TIP: Try this with different types of lentils. However, brown or green lentils will need additional cooking time, at least 15 more minutes.

Per Serving: Calories: 415; Total fat: 7g; Saturated fat: 1g; Sodium: 410mg; Carbohydrates: 67g; Fiber: 12g; Sugar: 5g; Protein: 24g

Sardine Salad

Dairy-Free, Gluten-Free, No Added Sugar, Nut-free, Omega-3-Rich, Soy-Free
Prep time: 10 minutes • **Serves 4**

Sardines are a shelf-stable, low-mercury, very high omega-3 fish, so they are an excellent, convenient, and healthy alternative to canned tuna (often high in inflammatory mercury). In this recipe, I use fermented pickles (I prefer the Bubbies brand) rather than relish; though it requires a few more minutes of prep, you will add probiotics and avoid artificial food colorings and sweeteners found in many relish brands. You can also replace the pickles with sauerkraut, if desired.

2 (4¼-ounce) cans sardines packed in olive oil, drained

¼ cup soy-free mayonnaise (I like the Sir Kensington's or Chosen Foods brands)

2 tablespoons Dijon mustard

2 tablespoons diced pickles

½ teaspoon dried dill

Freshly ground black pepper

2 scallions, white and green parts, chopped (optional)

Bread, mini sweet peppers, cucumber slices, or veggie dippers, for serving

1. Put the drained sardines in a medium bowl and mash with a fork. Stir in the mayonnaise, mustard, pickles, dill, pepper, and scallions (if using).

2. Serve on bread, in lettuce cups, stuffed into mini sweet peppers, on top of cucumber slices, or with veggie dippers such as carrot or celery sticks.

3. Store leftovers covered in the refrigerator for up to 5 days.

VARIATION TIP: To make one of my favorite variations—what I call Confetti Sardine Salad—add half a Granny Smith apple, chopped, and 2 tablespoons shredded carrots. The colors, sweetness, extra nutrition, and crunch add a nice complexity to the recipe.

Per Serving (¼ cup): Calories: 122; Total fat: 10g; Saturated fat: 1g; Sodium: 235mg; Carbohydrates: 1g; Fiber: 0g; Sugar: 0g; Protein: 7g

Easy Avocado Boiled Egg Salad

Dairy-Free, Gluten-Free, No Added Sugar, Nut-free, Omega-3-Rich, Soy-Free, Vegetarian
Prep time: 5 minutes, plus 5 minutes to chill / **Cook time:** 20 minutes • **Serves** 4

Filling avocado skins is a fun and resourceful way to avoid washing extra dishes. To make this a heartier meal, add 1 drained 15-ounce can of chickpeas to the salad before serving. Add extra lemon juice, salt, and pepper to taste. It won't all fit in the avocado shells, though! Eggs from pastured hens and the fats in the avocado will help increase the absorption of the anti-inflammatory nutrient *lycopene* in the tomatoes.

6 large eggs

1 avocado

1 cup halved cherry tomatoes

1 tablespoon freshly squeezed lemon juice

Sea salt

Freshly ground black pepper

1. Fill a large saucepan with water and add the eggs. Bring to a rolling boil, then remove from the heat and cover for 14 minutes.

2. Halve the avocado lengthwise and remove the pit. Carefully dice the flesh, scoop it out of the peels, and transfer it to a medium bowl.

3. Remove the eggs from the hot water and place in an ice bath for 5 minutes to cool. Peel the eggs, and chop.

4. Add the eggs, cherry tomatoes, lemon juice, salt, and pepper to the diced avocado. Gently stir. Scoop the egg salad into the empty avocado skins and serve.

5. Store leftovers in a sealed container in the refrigerator for up to 2 days.

VARIATION TIP: For a touch of spice, sprinkle cayenne pepper or replace the salt with Tajín seasoning—a Mexican seasoning available worldwide—that contains a combination of mild chiles, lime, and salt.

Per Serving (1 cup): Calories: 195; Total fat: 15g; Saturated fat: 3g; Sodium: 151mg; Carbohydrates: 7g; Fiber: 4g; Sugar: 2g; Protein: 11g

Warm Garlic Greens

Gluten-Free, No Added Sugar, Soy-Free, Vegan
Prep time: 5 minutes / **Cook time:** 15 minutes • **Serves 4**

According to abundant research, dark-leafy greens are one of the most important foods we can eat regularly. They are low in calories yet loaded with nutrients and beneficial compounds that help improve biomarkers, reduce inflammation, and decrease the risk of cancer, heart disease, and premature brain aging. Although you can use any mixed greens here, I love the combination of mustard, turnip, and collard greens. To create a full meal, pair with simple fried eggs, Easy Avocado Boiled Egg Salad (page 54), or Mushroom Beef Flax Meatballs (page 111).

1 tablespoon extra-virgin olive oil

2 tablespoons chopped red onion

4 cups prewashed, pre-chopped mixed leafy greens

2 garlic cloves, minced and set aside for 10 minutes

1 teaspoon apple cider vinegar

1 teaspoon Dijon mustard

Sea salt

Freshly ground black pepper

Roasted, salted pumpkin seeds (optional)

Chipotle chili powder or red pepper flakes (optional)

1. Heat the olive oil in a large nonstick skillet over medium heat. Sauté the onion for 2 to 3 minutes, then add the chopped greens. Stir occasionally and cook until the greens are soft and wilted, 4 to 6 minutes. Add the garlic and sauté for 1 to 2 more minutes to soften. Stir in the vinegar and mustard and remove from the heat. Taste and add more vinegar, salt, and pepper as needed.

2. Sprinkle with salted pumpkin seeds (if using), or chipotle chili powder/red pepper flakes (if using).

Per Serving: Calories: 42; Total fat: 4g; Saturated fat: 0g; Sodium: 56mg; Carbohydrates: 2g; Fiber: 1g; Sugar: 1g; Protein: 1g

Watermelon and Quinoa Salad with Feta and Mint

Gluten-Free, Nut-Free, No Added Sugar, Soy-Free, Vegetarian
Prep time: 10 minutes / **Cook time:** 25 minutes • **Serves** 4

This salad screams summer. The quinoa adds protein and fiber, and the watermelon is sweet, juicy, and a delicious counterpart to the creamy feta. Because most markets sell cut watermelon, this salad is a breeze to create. I also love to replace the watermelon with fresh peaches.

2 cups water

1 cup quinoa, rinsed

1 teaspoon salt

¼ cup extra-virgin olive oil

2 tablespoons freshly squeezed
   lemon juice

2 cups seeded watermelon, cut into
   ½-inch dice

½ cup crumbled sheep's or goat's milk
   feta cheese

¼ cup finely chopped fresh mint

¼ teaspoon freshly ground black pepper

1. In a large stockpot, combine the water, quinoa, and salt. Bring to a boil over medium-high heat, reduce to low, and simmer, partially covered, until all the water has been absorbed, 15 to 20 minutes. Remove from the heat, let cool to room temperature, and fluff with a fork.

2. Add the oil and lemon juice and mix well.

3. Add the watermelon and gently mix until just combined.

4. Sprinkle the cheese, mint, and pepper over the salad and serve.

PREP TIP: If using cooked quinoa, use 3 cups. This salad is best eaten shortly after it's been made but can be refrigerated, covered, for 24 hours.

Per Serving: Calories: 353; Total fat: 20g; Saturated fat: 5g; Sodium: 698mg; Carbohydrates: 35g; Fiber: 4g; Sugar: 6g; Protein: 9g

Chickpea and Kale Salad

Dairy-Free, Gluten-Free, No Added Sugar, Nut-Free, Soy-Free, Vegan
Prep time: 10 minutes / **Cook time:** 20 minutes • **Serves 4**

I know what you're thinking: *Raw kale is not for me.* Hold that thought. The secret to eating and enjoying kale raw is giving it a good massage with olive oil, lemon juice, and salt first. This helps wilt and break down the greens so they're more palatable and easier to digest. Once you give kale some love, it will love you right back with its wonderful taste and healthy nutrients.

1 large bunch kale, thoroughly washed, stemmed, and cut into thin strips
2 tablespoons extra-virgin olive oil, divided
2 teaspoons freshly squeezed lemon juice

¾ teaspoon salt, divided
2 cups cooked chickpeas
1 teaspoon sweet paprika
1 avocado, chopped (optional)

1. In a large bowl, combine the kale, 1 tablespoon oil, the lemon juice, and ¼ teaspoon salt. With your hands, massage the kale for 5 minutes, or until it starts to wilt and becomes bright green and shiny.

2. Heat the remaining 1 tablespoon of oil in a large skillet on medium-low heat. Add the chickpeas, paprika, and remaining ½ teaspoon of salt. Cook for about 15 minutes or until warm. The chickpeas might start to crisp in spots.

3. Pour the chickpeas over the kale. Toss well. Add the avocado (if using). Serve immediately.

VARIATION TIP: If you don't want to use paprika, try other herbs and spices. Dried basil, oregano, dill, parsley, garlic or onion powder, cumin, chili powder, or turmeric work well. You can also omit the herbs and just use salt.

Per Serving: Calories: 204; Total fat: 9g; Saturated fat: 1g; Sodium: 448mg; Carbohydrates: 24g; Fiber: 7g; Sugar: 4g; Protein: 8g

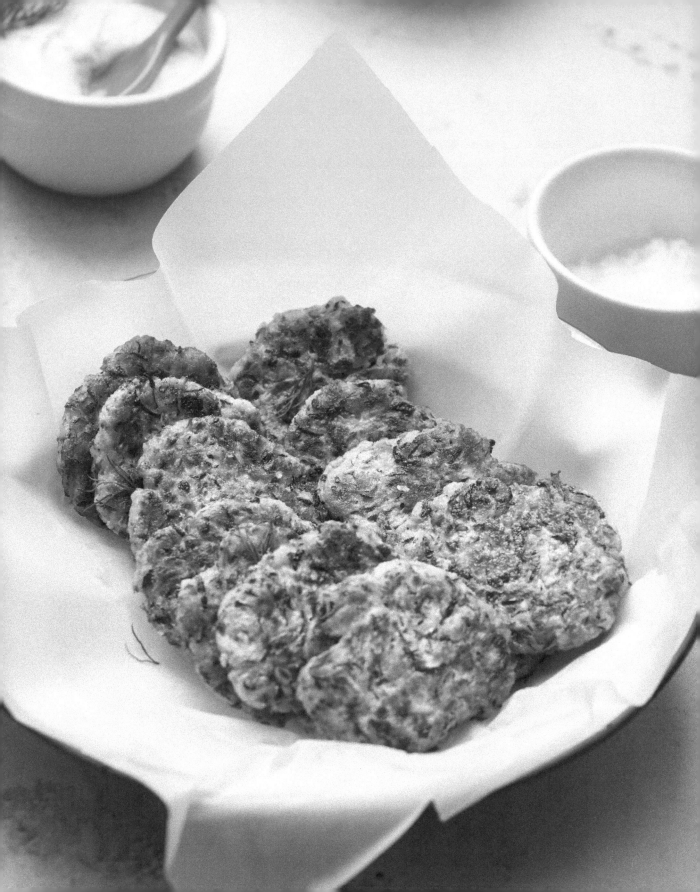

CHAPTER 5

VEGETARIAN MAINS

Stuffed Sweet Potatoes

Gluten-Free, No Added Sugar, Soy-Free, Vegetarian
Prep time: 5 minutes / **Cook time:** 57 minutes • **Serves** 4

This recipe is a powerhouse meal packed with anti-inflammatory carotenoids, antioxidants, probiotics, fiber, and plant protein. Busy people everywhere rejoice: Although the cook time is longer than most recipes in this cookbook, it's largely inactive time, so you can still multitask. Another option to speed up dinnertime is to make the potatoes ahead of time, refrigerate until ready, and reheat in the oven or microwave.

4 medium sweet potatoes
1 (15-ounce) can low-sodium black beans, drained and rinsed
1 cup water
2 cups fresh baby spinach

¼ cup hot sauce (I like Frank's RedHot Original Buffalo Sauce)
½ cup full-fat or low-fat Greek yogurt
½ teaspoon salt
½ teaspoon freshly ground black pepper

1. Preheat the oven to 400°F. Wash the sweet potatoes, dry, then wrap each individually in foil. Bake for 50 minutes or until soft when squeezed.

2. Meanwhile, in a small saucepan, warm the black beans and water over medium-low heat for about 5 minutes. Alternatively, you may skip this step and proceed with room-temperature beans.

3. Once cooked, slice each potato lengthwise, only halfway down so as not to tear the bottom skin layer. Lightly squeeze both ends to soften the flesh. Add ½ cup spinach to each potato, then squeeze the sides to reseal for about 2 minutes to soften the greens. Reopen the potatoes and top each with 1 tablespoon of hot sauce, 2 tablespoons of yogurt, salt, and pepper.

PREP TIP: To save time: Fill a pressure cooker with 1 inch of water and add your steamer basket. Put 4 washed sweet potatoes in the basket, lock the lid, and pressure cook on high for 12 minutes, then natural release for 10 minutes.

Per Serving (1 potato): Calories: 221; Total fat: 1g; Saturated fat: 0g; Sodium: 487mg; Carbohydrates: 44g; Fiber: 10g; Sugar: 8g; Protein: 10g

Walnut Bean Burgers

Gluten-Free, No Added Sugar, Omega-3-Rich, Soy-Free, Vegan
Prep time: 10 minutes / **Cook time:** 25 minutes • **Serves 4**

Incorporating beans in patty form is an excellent way to boost your fiber, anti-oxidants, and gut-nourishing nutrients. Replace the black beans with any firm canned bean you fancy. The walnuts add texture and omega-3s. Can't find adobo seasoning? Use an all-purpose seasoning of your choice. Some seasonings contain much more sodium than others. I like to serve these on a bed of spinach, with tomato, avocado, jalapeño, chipotle sauce, and/or Dijon mustard.

¼ cup shredded carrots

¼ onion, any color

2 tablespoons chopped walnuts

1 tablespoon extra-virgin olive oil

1–2 teaspoons adobo seasoning (see headnote)

1 garlic clove, minced (optional)

1 tablespoon hot sauce (optional)

1 (15-ounce) can low-sodium black beans, drained and rinsed

1. Preheat the oven to 400°F. Line a baking sheet with parchment paper.

2. In a food processor bowl, combine the carrots, onion, walnuts, oil, seasoning, garlic (if using), and hot sauce (if using). Pulse until evenly mixed and onions are minced. Then add the black beans and pulse once or twice to incorporate. You want to still see pieces of black bean.

3. Scoop about ¼ cup of the mixture onto the baking sheet and press lightly to make a patty shape. Repeat with the remaining mixture until all the patties are formed. The mixture will be soft and moist. They will firm up in the oven the longer they bake.

4. Bake for about 10 minutes, flip, then bake for another 10 minutes. When the patties are firm enough to pick up, they are done. Be careful not to overbake them, or they will be dry and crumbly.

Per Serving (1 burger): Calories: 148; Total fat: 6g; Saturated fat: 1g; Sodium: 300mg; Carbohydrates: 18g; Fiber: 6g; Sugar: 1g; Protein: 7g

Pesto Lentil Pasta

Gluten-Free, No Added Sugar, Nut-free, Omega-3-Rich, Soy-Free, Vegetarian
Prep time: 15 minutes / **Cook time:** 20 minutes • **Serves** 4

This is a lighter, fresher, and gut-healthier version of a traditional pasta dish. Green or red lentil pasta is not only high-fiber and high-protein, but it's also gluten-free and more filling than refined wheat-based pastas. Pea pasta is also an excellent substitute; I love the ZENB brand. Pine nuts (actually seeds from pine cones and not nuts at all) can be enjoyed by those with nut allergies. Pumpkin seeds are also an easy swap.

8 ounces lentil pasta (any shape)

3 garlic cloves

1 tablespoon extra-virgin olive oil

2 tablespoons chopped walnuts

1 cup cherry tomatoes

2 cups baby spinach

¼ cup basil pesto

½ teaspoon salt

½ teaspoon freshly ground black pepper

1. Cook the pasta in a large saucepan according to the package directions and reserve 1 cup cooking water before draining the pasta. Set the pasta aside.

2. While the pasta is cooking, mince the garlic and set aside for 10 minutes.

3. Heat the oil in the same large saucepan over medium heat and sauté the garlic and walnuts for 1 to 2 minutes. Add the tomatoes and cook until blistered, 3 to 4 minutes. Add the spinach and cook for 2 minutes to wilt it. Reduce the heat to medium-low.

4. Add the cooked pasta and pesto and cook for 2 to 3 minutes. Add the reserved pasta water, 1 tablespoon at a time, stirring until the pasta appears saucier, or to your liking. Season with salt and pepper to taste.

VARIATION TIP: For dairy-free pesto: In a small processor, puree 1 cup basil, the juice from ½ lemon, 2 tablespoons pine nuts or pumpkin seeds, 1 garlic clove, 3 tablespoons olive oil, ¼ teaspoon salt, and 1 tablespoon nutritional yeast. Refrigerate for up to a week.

Per Serving: Calories: 265; Total fat: 7g; Saturated fat: 1g; Sodium: 310mg; Carbohydrates: 46g; Fiber: 6 g; Sugar: 1g; Protein: 10g

Sheet Pan Winter Vegetable Bake

Dairy-Free, Gluten-Free, Nut-Free, Soy-Free, Vegetarian
Prep time: 10 minutes / **Cook time:** 35 minutes • **Serves** 4

This is an easy, all-in-one, versatile, nutrient-rich, and anti-inflammatory recipe. For the vegetables, empty your produce drawer or look for a prepared mix at your market that contains beets, carrots, sweet potatoes, and/or parsnips. Alternatively, you can replace it with your choice of winter squash, Brussels sprouts, or just one of the options above. Feel free to replace the canned lentils with canned chickpeas or with 1 cup of potatoes if you prefer—the sky's the limit!

1 red onion, quartered

2 cups chopped root vegetables

1 cup halved cherry tomatoes

2 tablespoons balsamic vinegar

1 tablespoon extra-virgin olive oil

1 tablespoon honey

1 tablespoon minced rosemary, oregano, or both (optional)

½ teaspoon salt

½ teaspoon freshly ground black pepper

1 (10½-ounce) can lentils, drained and rinsed (optional)

1. Preheat the oven to 400°F. Line a sheet pan with parchment paper.

2. Spread the onion, root vegetables, and tomatoes on the prepared sheet pan and toss with the vinegar, oil, honey, herbs (if using), salt, and pepper and mix well.

3. Bake for 40 to 45 minutes, stirring the vegetables halfway through to ensure even cooking. If using lentils, add them the last 10 minutes of baking.

PREP TIP: Produce and freezer sections often have a variety of "steamer bags" that contain pre-washed, pre-chopped produce. This is an excellent place to look to save vegetable prep time for your recipes.

Per Serving (1 cup): Calories: 96; Total fat: 4g; Saturated fat: 1g; Sodium: 338mg; Carbohydrates: 16g; Fiber: 3g; Sugar: 10g; Protein: 1g

Chipotle Cauliflower Bowl

Dairy-Free, Gluten-Free, No Added Sugar, Nut-free, Soy-Free, Vegan
Prep time: 8 minutes / **Cook time:** 8 minutes • **Serves** 4 (about 1½ cups)

Smoky, spicy, healthy fats, high-fiber, and cruciferous vegetables—this recipe makes an all-in-one plant-based meal or a lovely side. My favorite brand of chipotle peppers is the San Marcos brand. Not a big spicy-food fan? Omit the pepper, and only use sauce from the can.

1 head cauliflower, stem removed, chopped into bite-size pieces

1 (16-ounce) can white beans, drained and rinsed

1 chipotle pepper in adobo and 1 tablespoon sauce (from a 7½-ounce can)

1 tablespoon water

2 teaspoons extra-virgin olive oil

Juice of 1 lime

½ teaspoon ground cumin (optional)

1 avocado, diced

1. In a medium saucepan with a steamer insert, bring an inch of water to a simmer over medium heat. Add the cauliflower, cover, and steam for 5 minutes. Add the beans on top to warm and steam for another 2 to 3 minutes or until the cauliflower is fork-tender.

2. Meanwhile, make the dressing. In a small food processor or blender, puree the pepper and sauce from the can, water, olive oil, lime juice, and cumin (if using) until creamy. Set aside.

3. To each bowl, spoon about 1 cup cauliflower, a heaping ⅓ cup of beans, and ¼ avocado. Drizzle the chipotle sauce on top. Enjoy.

VARIATION TIP: You can replace the cauliflower with kale or other hardy leafy green for a different flavor profile or if you just want to use up vegetables that you have on hand.

Per Serving: Calories: 236; Total fat: 10g; Saturated fat: 2g; Sodium: 49mg; Carbohydrates: 30g; Fiber: 13g; Sugar: 3g; Protein: 10g

Grain-Free Fritters

Dairy-Free, Gluten-Free, No Added Sugar, Soy-Free, Vegan
Prep time: 5 minutes / **Cook time:** 20 minutes • **Makes** 12 fritters

These grain-free fritters are easy to make, hold together well, and have a surprisingly eggy flavor. There are two keys to their success: Use medium-low heat to cook the fritters gently and evenly, and don't flip them too soon. After dolloping the batter into the skillet, resist the instinct to slide the spatula under the fritters to "check if they're sticking." Pair with a simple spinach salad for a light lunch or dinner, or dip into a mixture of plain yogurt and lemon juice.

2 cups chickpea flour

1½ cups water

2 tablespoons chia seeds, ground

1 teaspoon sweet paprika

2 garlic cloves, minced

½ teaspoon salt

3 cups lightly packed spinach leaves, finely chopped

1 tablespoon coconut oil or extra-virgin olive oil

1. In a medium bowl, whisk together the chickpea flour, water, chia seeds, paprika, garlic, and salt. Mix well to ensure there are no lumps. Fold in the spinach.

2. In a large nonstick skillet over medium-low heat, melt the coconut oil. Working in batches, use a ¼-cup measure to drop the batter into the pan. Flatten the fritters to about ½-inch thick. Don't crowd the skillet.

3. Cook for 5 to 6 minutes, flip, and cook for 5 minutes more. Serve warm.

VARIATION TIP: Any dark leafy green can be substituted cup for cup for the spinach. Also try broccoli, zucchini, carrots, and sweet potatoes or add extra spices such as ground ginger, cumin, turmeric, coriander, dried basil, oregano, or rosemary.

Per Serving (2 fritters): Calories: 318; Total fat: 10g; Saturated fat: 1g; Sodium: 222mg; Carbohydrates: 45g; Fiber: 15g; Sugar: 7g; Protein: 15g

Spiced Broccoli, Cauliflower, and Tofu

Gluten-Free, No Added Sugar, Soy-Free, Vegan
Prep time: 10 minutes / **Cook time:** 25 minutes • **Serves 4**

Many markets sell prepackaged broccoli and cauliflower florets, which eliminates the need to cut the vegetables. Roasting cruciferous vegetables will make them more enticing to people who don't love cruciferous vegetables, as it removes much of their bitter taste.

4 cups broccoli-cauliflower mix (thawed, if frozen)
1 medium red onion, diced
3 tablespoons extra-virgin olive oil
1 teaspoon salt
¼ teaspoon freshly ground black pepper

1 pound firm tofu, drained, cut into 1-inch cubes
2 garlic cloves, minced
1 (½-inch) piece fresh ginger, peeled and minced

1. Preheat the oven to 400°F.

2. On a large baking sheet, combine the broccoli, cauliflower, onion, oil, salt, and pepper and mix well.

3. Transfer the baking sheet to the oven and roast until the vegetables have softened, 10 to 15 minutes. Meanwhile, press the tofu between paper towels to remove as much moisture as you can.

4. Add the tofu, garlic, and ginger.

5. Return the baking sheet to the oven and roast until the vegetables are tender and the tofu is lightly browned, about 10 minutes.

6. Gently mix the ingredients on the baking sheet to combine the tofu with the vegetables and serve.

VARIATION TIP: If you're avoiding soy, you can make this dish with canned beans or cooked chicken. Store, covered, in the refrigerator for up to 5 days, or freeze for several months.

Per Serving: Calories: 210; Total fat: 15g; Saturated fat: 1g; Sodium: 626mg; Carbohydrates: 11g; Fiber: 4g; Sugar: 4g; Protein: 12g

Quinoa Flatbread Pizza

Gluten-Free, Nut-Free, Soy-Free, Vegetarian

Prep time: 10 minutes, plus 8 hours to soak / **Cook time:** 40 minutes • **Makes** 1 (8-inch) thick-crust flatbread, or 2 thin crusts

The quinoa flatbread base used in this recipe is going to become your favorite gluten-free pizza crust of all time. It's thin yet hearty and stands up well to toppings. What I use here are some simple topping suggestions. If you've got more vegetables, herbs, or proteins in the refrigerator that need to be used, pile them on. This crust can take it.

¾ cup dry quinoa, rinsed

1¾ cups water, divided

½ teaspoon baking powder

½ teaspoon salt

2 tablespoons extra-virgin olive oil, divided

1 cup marinara or pasta sauce

1 cup sliced mushrooms

2 cups arugula

1 teaspoon red pepper flakes (optional)

6 slices fresh mozzarella or ½ cup shredded (optional)

1. In a glass container, combine the quinoa and 1½ cups water and soak for 8 hours or overnight. Rinse and drain.

2. Preheat the oven to 425°F. Line a 9-inch round cake pan or pie pan (or two pans for two thin crusts) with parchment paper.

3. In a blender, combine the quinoa, the remaining ¼ cup water, the baking powder, the salt, and 1 tablespoon oil and blend until creamy.

4. Pour the mixture into the prepared pan. If making 1 thick crust, bake for 20 minutes, flip, and then bake for another 10 minutes before removing for toppings. If making two thin crusts, bake for 20 minutes, then remove for toppings.

5. Remove the pan, brush the crust with the remaining 1 tablespoon olive oil, and add toppings of marinara, mushrooms, arugula, and red pepper flakes (if using). Tear and scatter the mozzarella (if using).

6. Put the pizza back in the oven and bake for 10 minutes. Cool the pizza slightly before slicing and serving.

PREP TIP: The crust can be made ahead of time. Allow it to cool completely and wrap tightly in parchment paper. Refrigerate if using in the next few days or place it in a resealable plastic freezer bag and freeze for another time.

Per Serving (¼ of thick pizza): Calories: 181; Total fat: 13g; Saturated fat: 2g; Sodium: 407mg; Carbohydrates: 13g; Fiber: 2g; Sugar: 2g; Protein: 4g

Baked Falafel

Gluten-Free, No Added Sugar, Nut-Free, Soy-Free, Vegan
Prep time: 15 minutes / **Cook time:** 30 minutes • **Makes 24 patties**

Falafel is traditionally deep-fried—usually in omega-6 oils at extremely high temperatures—which can contribute to inflammation. This recipe is baked, creating a much healthier and easier option because the cooking is hands-off.

3 cups cooked chickpeas
⅓ cup tahini
1 tablespoon ground cumin
4 garlic cloves

½ teaspoon salt
½ bunch parsley, chopped
1 tablespoon lemon juice (optional)
Water, for thinning

1. Preheat the oven to 350°F. Line a baking sheet with parchment paper.

2. In a food processor, combine the chickpeas, tahini, cumin, garlic, and salt. Process until mostly smooth. Add the parsley and lemon juice (if using) and pulse until incorporated. If necessary, add 1 or 2 tablespoons of water to help the ingredients form a ball, being careful not to add too much. The mixture should not be wet and pasty.

3. Measure 2 tablespoons of dough, roll it into a ball, and place it on the baking sheet. With the bottom of a glass or using your hand, press the ball into a patty about 1 inch thick. Repeat with the remaining chickpea mixture; it should yield about 24 patties.

4. Bake for 30 minutes. The falafels will be quite soft when straight out of the oven, but they firm as they cool.

PREP TIP: A spring-loaded ice cream scoop is an incredibly handy kitchen tool. It's great for scooping ice cream, of course, but it also creates uniform falafels, burger patties, muffins, and cookies. This helps food cook evenly. I use both a 1-ounce and 3-ounce scooper regularly for various kitchen tasks.

Per Serving (2 balls): Calories: 111; Total fat: 5g; Saturated fat: 1g; Sodium: 110mg; Carbohydrates: 13g; Fiber: 4g; Sugar: 2g; Protein: 5g

Vegetable Spring Roll Wraps

Dairy-Free, Gluten-Free, No Added Sugar, Nut-Free, Soy-Free, Vegan
Prep time: 20 minutes • **Makes** 10 wraps

This recipe is great for when you crave something light and fresh, or when it's just too hot to cook. Rice paper wrappers can be found in most international sections of grocery stores. These wrappers need to be soaked in warm water for a minute or two to become pliable. The first time you use them, it might take a roll or two before you perfect your wrapping technique.

2 cups lightly packed baby spinach

1 cup grated carrot, divided

1 cucumber, halved, seeded, and cut into thin, 4-inch-long strips, divided

1 avocado, halved, pitted, and cut into thin strips, divided

10 rice paper wrappers

Tamari sauce for dipping (optional)

1. Spread the spinach, carrot, cucumber, and avocado on a flat surface.

2. Fill a large, shallow bowl with warm water, hot enough to cook the wrappers but cool enough so you can touch the water comfortably.

3. Soak 1 wrapper in the water and then place it on the cutting board.

4. Arrange ¼ cup of spinach, 2 tablespoons of grated carrot, a few cucumber slices, and 1 or 2 slices of avocado in the middle of the wrapper.

5. Fold the sides over the middle, and then roll the wrapper tightly from the bottom (the side closest to you), burrito-style.

6. Repeat with the remaining wrappers and vegetables. Serve immediately with tamari sauce (if using).

PREP TIP: If not serving right away, the rice paper wrappers will dry out within 1 hour. To prevent this, lightly dampen a paper towel or cloth napkin and cover the rolls to keep them moist.

Per Serving (2 rolls): Calories: 246; Total fat: 10g; Saturated fat: 1g; Sodium: 145mg; Carbohydrates: 36g; Fiber: 6g; Sugar: 4g; Protein: 4g

Buckwheat-Vegetable Polenta

Dairy-Free, Gluten-Free, No Added Sugar, Nut-Free, Soy-Free, Vegan
Prep time: 15 minutes / **Cook time:** 20 minutes • **Serves 6**

Miss creamy polenta? You won't when buckwheat is around. This special, magnesium-rich fruit seed has a consistency like polenta when ground into meal. This vegetable polenta isn't "traditional," but it is delicious.

3 cups buckwheat

¼ cup extra-virgin olive oil

6 garlic cloves, minced

6 cups warm vegetable broth

2 cups shredded zucchini

6 cups spinach, finely chopped

1 teaspoon salt, plus additional as needed

1. In a spice grinder, high-speed blender, or food processor, pulse the buck-wheat until finely ground.

2. In a large saucepan on medium-low heat, heat the olive oil. Add the garlic and sauté for 3 minutes. Add the ground buckwheat and stir to coat.

3. Stir in 1 cup of vegetable broth. When all the liquid is absorbed, add another cup of broth, along with the zucchini and spinach. Repeat with the remaining 4 cups of broth, 1 cup at a time, until the buckwheat is tender and the consistency of a thick polenta. You may not need to use all the broth. Add the salt, stir, taste, and adjust the seasoning if necessary.

VARIATION TIP: If you and your dinner mates are not vegetarian, use chicken broth instead. You can even make this recipe with plain water, but you might need to add some additional salt and herbs for flavor.

Per Serving: Calories: 426; Total fat: 13g; Saturated fat: 1g; Sodium: 647mg; Carbohydrates: 65g; Fiber: 10g; Sugar: 2g; Protein: 18g

Tahini Kale Noodles

Dairy-Free, Gluten-Free, No Added Sugar, Vegan
Prep time: 5 minutes / **Cook time:** 8 to 10 minutes • **Serves 4**

What constitutes the right cooking volume of pasta or noodles? Grab a fistful of noodles between the size of a dime's diameter (1 ounce dry) and a quarter's (2 ounces dry). This recipe is a powerhouse of anti-inflammatory nutrients including amino acids and vitamins C and A and includes a payload of calcium.

8 ounces lentil spaghetti or buckwheat noodles
4 cups lightly packed baby kale or
  chopped kale
½ cup tahini
¾ cup hot water, plus additional as needed

¼ teaspoon salt, plus additional as needed
½ cup chopped fresh parsley
Juice of 1 lemon
1 tablespoon nutritional yeast (optional)
2 scallions, green and white parts, sliced
  (optional)

1. Cook the noodles according to the package instructions. During the last 30 seconds of cook time, toss in the kale. In a colander, drain the noodles and kale. Transfer to a large bowl.

2. In a medium bowl, stir together the tahini, hot water, and salt. If you'd like a thinner sauce, add more water.

3. Add the parsley, lemon juice, sauce, and nutritional yeast (if using) to the noodles and toss to coat. Taste, and adjust the seasoning if necessary. Top with scallions (if using) and serve hot or cold.

VARIATION TIP: Not into tahini? Use sunflower seed butter, pumpkin seed butter, almond butter, walnut butter, or cashew butter instead.

Per Serving: Calories: 404; Total fat: 18g; Saturated fat: 2g; Sodium: 223mg; Carbohydrates: 54g; Fiber: 10g; Sugar: 2g; Protein: 15g

Broccoli and Bean Casserole

Dairy-Free, Gluten-Free, Omega-3-Rich, Soy-Free, Vegan
Prep time: 10 minutes / **Cook time:** 35 to 40 minutes • **Serves** 4

Don't toss out those broccoli stalks. They contain nutrients similar to those in the florets, and they taste the same, too. You can freeze them to use later when making soup or stock. This recipe calls for a bean seasoning blend, but I also love Bragg's All-Purpose Seasoning. If your seasoning is unsalted, add about 1 teaspoon of salt. I love eating this with fried eggs and salsa.

¾ cup water or vegetable broth

2 medium broccoli heads, crowns and stalks finely chopped

2 teaspoons borracho/pinto bean seasoning (or all-purpose seasoning blend)

½ teaspoon salt

1½ cups cooked pinto or navy beans, or 1 (14-ounce) can, drained

1 to 2 tablespoons brown rice flour or arrowroot flour

2 teaspoons nutritional yeast (optional)

1 cup walnuts, chopped

¼ cup salsa (optional)

1. Preheat the oven to 350°F.

2. In a large ovenproof pot set on medium heat, warm the water. Add the broccoli, seasoning mix, and salt and cook for 6 to 8 minutes, or until the broccoli is bright green.

3. Stir in the beans, brown rice flour, and nutritional yeast (if using). Cook for 5 minutes more, or until the liquid thickens slightly. Sprinkle the walnuts over the top.

4. Bake for 20 to 25 minutes. The walnuts should be toasted. Serve with your favorite salsa if desired.

VARIATION TIP: For nut-free, use sunflower seeds or pumpkin seeds to replace the walnuts. Not dairy-free? Replace the nutritional yeast with ¼ cup shredded sharp cheddar. Add it on top during the last 10 minutes of baking to create a cheesy top.

Per Serving: Calories: 410; Total fat: 20g; Saturated fat: 3g; Sodium: 535mg; Carbohydrates: 43g; Fiber: 13g; Sugar: 4g; Protein: 22g

Homemade Avocado Sushi

Gluten-Free, Soy-Free, Vegan
Prep time: 20 minutes / **Cook time:** 15 minutes • **Serves 4**

This take on sushi is easy to make at home, and you don't need any unique equipment such as bamboo mats or chopsticks. The only special ingredient you'll need is nori sheets, which are readily available nowadays in the international section of most supermarkets. Traditionally, sushi is prepared with white rice; here, I use quinoa for superior nutrition and a lower blood sugar response. The sky is the limit on your ability to customize this—try adding matchstick jalapeños, carrots, scallions, and more.

3 cups water, plus additional for rolling
1½ cups dry quinoa, rinsed
½ teaspoon salt
6 nori sheets
3 avocados, halved, pitted, and sliced
  thin, divided

1 small cucumber, halved, seeded, and cut
  into matchsticks, divided
Tamari or coconut aminos, for dipping
  (optional)

1. In a medium saucepan set over high heat, combine the water, quinoa, and salt and bring to a boil. Reduce the heat to low, cover, and simmer for 15 minutes. Remove from the heat, fluff the quinoa with a fork, and set aside.

2. On a cutting board, lay out 1 nori sheet. Spread ½ cup of quinoa over the sheet, leaving 2 to 3 inches uncovered at the top.

3. Place 5 or 6 avocado slices across the bottom of the nori sheet (the side closest to you) in a row. Add 5 or 6 cucumber matchsticks on top.

4. Starting at the bottom, tightly roll up the nori sheet. Dab the uncovered top with water to seal the roll.

5. Slice the sushi roll into 6 pieces.

continued >>

6. Repeat with the remaining 5 nori sheets, quinoa, and vegetables.

7. Serve with tamari, if using.

VARIATION TIP: Coconut aminos, derived from coconuts, mimics the taste of soy sauce but is naturally sweeter. It can be difficult to locate and is often expensive. Another option for dipping is tahini.

Per Serving: Calories: 557; Total fat: 33g; Saturated fat: 4g; Sodium: 309mg; Carbohydrates: 57g; Fiber: 5g; Sugar: 2g; Protein: 13g

One-Pot Mushroom Pasta

Gluten-Free, Nut-Free, Soy-Free, Vegan
Prep time: 15 minutes / **Cook time:** 20 minutes • **Serves 4**

As crazy as it sounds, in this recipe the pasta and sauce cook together. That way the pasta absorbs the mushroom juices, creating a flavorful, satisfying dish—and with one less pot to worry about. A generous dusting of grated Parmesan cheese is the perfect way to finish off this dish if you don't need it to be vegetarian or vegan.

2 tablespoons extra-virgin olive oil, plus more for drizzling

2 cups quartered button or cremini mushrooms

¼ cup dry red or white wine

1 teaspoon salt

¼ teaspoon freshly ground black pepper

1 shallot, minced

1 garlic clove, minced

4 to 4½ cups water

1 (12-ounce) package pea or lentil rigatoni

1 teaspoon nutritional yeast (optional)

1 teaspoon chopped fresh rosemary (optional)

1. Heat the olive oil in a large saucepan with a lid or Dutch oven over high heat. Once hot, add the mushrooms, wine, salt, and pepper. Sauté until the mushrooms are cooked, about 5 minutes. Add the shallot and garlic and stir to combine. Cook for 1 more minute.

2. Add 4 cups of water and the rigatoni and bring to a boil. Reduce to a simmer, cover, and cook until the pasta is tender and most of the water is absorbed, 12 to 15 minutes.

3. If the mixture is too thick, add up to ½ cup more water. Transfer to a serving bowl, stir in the nutritional yeast (if using), drizzle with olive oil, top with the rosemary (if using), and serve.

4. This dish can be refrigerated for up to a week, then reheated and served.

VARIATION TIP: If you're not avoiding gluten, you can substitute whole wheat pasta. Need to minimize fiber for a digestive condition? Brown rice or corn pasta work great.

Per Serving: Calories: 350; Total fat: 6g; Saturated fat: 0g; Sodium: 580mg; Carbohydrates: 58g; Fiber: 10g; Sugar: 3g; Protein: 19g

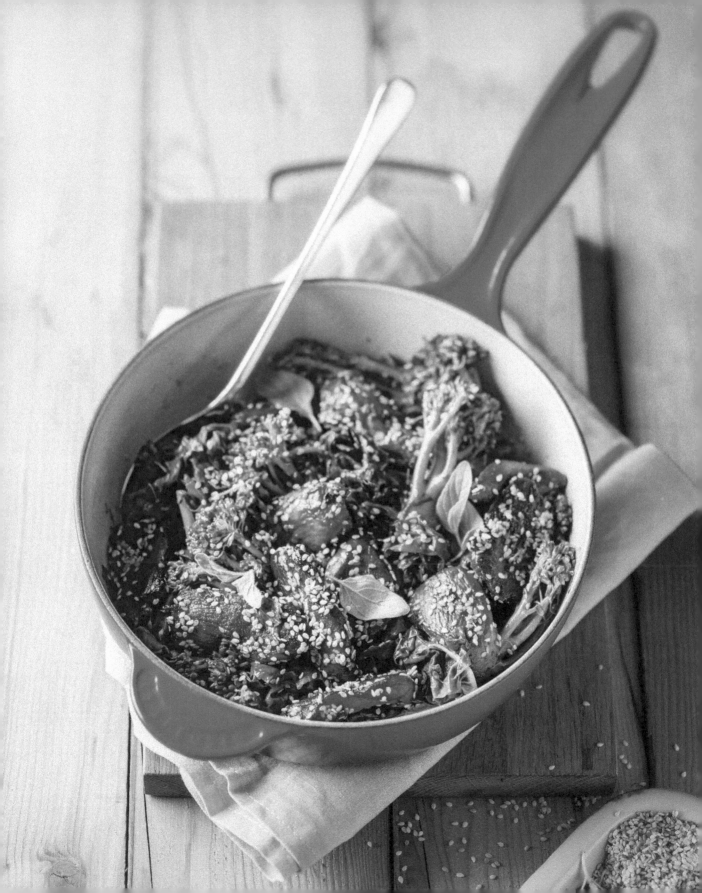

CHAPTER 6

POULTRY AND SEAFOOD

One-Pan Pesto and Artichoke Chicken

Dairy-Free, Gluten-Free, No Added Sugar, Soy-Free
Prep time: 10 minutes / **Cook time:** 20 minutes · **Serves 4**

When you're tired, worn out, or not feeling good, a healthy, yummy dinner with easy cleanup is worth gold. This dinner has prebiotic fiber from artichokes, and antioxidants from olives, tomatoes, and pesto. It's also low in carbs to minimize blood sugar spikes. This recipe works great for meal prep, so you can make it ahead and refrigerate it for up to 5 days. Check out the variation tip in the Pesto Lentil Pasta (page 62) for a quick dairy-free pesto.

1 pound boneless, skinless chicken breasts
1 tablespoon extra-virgin olive oil
½ teaspoon salt
½ ground black pepper
16 ounces frozen artichoke hearts, thawed

1 cup cherry tomatoes
¼ cup kalamata olives
2 tablespoons water
⅓ cup basil pesto
Juice of 1 lemon (optional)

1. Preheat the oven to 350°F.

2. Heat a large cast-iron skillet over medium-high heat. Brush the chicken breasts with olive oil and season with salt and pepper. Sear the chicken for 3 to 4 minutes on each side. The chicken will loosen from the pan when it's ready to be flipped. Remove the skillet from the heat.

3. Add the artichoke hearts, tomatoes, and olives evenly around the chicken. Drizzle the water, any remaining olive oil from basting, and the pesto on top.

4. Bake for 10 to 12 minutes or until the chicken reaches an internal temperature of 165°F. Squeeze fresh lemon on top (if using) before serving.

Per Serving: Calories: 213; Total fat: 7g; Saturated fat: 1g; Sodium: 466mg; Carbohydrates: 11g; Fiber: 5g; Sugar: 1g; Protein: 29g

Grilled Five-Spice Chicken Skewers

Dairy-Free, Gluten-Free
Prep time: 15 minutes, plus 30 minutes to chill / **Cook time:** 20 minutes • **Makes 8 skewers**

Five-spice seasoning typically contains cinnamon, fennel, cloves, star anise, and white pepper. It's reminiscent of Jamaican jerk seasoning but is often used in Asian cuisine. Replace it with jerk seasoning if you prefer. I love to serve these skewers with sautéed bok choy or steamed broccoli for a boost of the sulfur-rich, anti-inflammatory, and anticancer compound sulforaphane. If you are using coconut aminos, it contains much less sodium than tamari or soy sauce, so sprinkle 1/2 teaspoon salt into the marinade. Don't have enough juice from the pineapple? Replace it with orange juice or minced pineapple.

1 tablespoon extra-virgin olive oil

1½ tablespoons five-spice blend

2 tablespoons tamari or coconut aminos

1 cup fresh pineapple, bite-size pieces, some juice reserved

1 pound boneless, skinless chicken thighs, cut into 1-inch pieces

½ red onion, chopped into large sections

16 garlic cloves (optional)

2 jalapeño peppers, quartered (optional)

1. In a casserole dish, combine the olive oil, five-spice blend, tamari, and 2 tablespoons of pineapple juice. Add the chicken, stir to evenly coat, and marinate in the refrigerator for 30 minutes.

2. Preheat the oven to 350°F.

3. Skewer the chicken, pineapple, onion, garlic (if using), and jalapeño (if using), in an alternating pattern until all ingredients are used (making 8 skewers). Reserve the marinade liquid.

continued >>

4. Preheat an outdoor grill (see tip) to medium-high heat. Place the skewers on the grill, brush with remaining marinade, and close the lid. Grill for about 8 minutes total, turning once or twice to prevent burning and ensure even cooking. Cool slightly, taste, sprinkle more five-spice, soy sauce, or tamari, if desired, then serve.

VARIATION TIP: If you'd rather not go outside to cook, you can use an indoor grill over medium heat, or bake the skewers in the oven on 400°F for about 10 to 12 minutes. Broil for another 2 to 3 minutes until the chicken is caramelized.

Per Serving (2 skewers): Calories: 201; Total fat: 8g; Saturated fat: 2g; Sodium: 502mg; Carbohydrates: 8g; Fiber: 1g; Sugar: 5g; Protein: 24g

Glazed Chicken with Broccoli

Dairy-Free, Gluten-Free, Soy-Free
Prep time: 15 minutes / **Cook time:** 35 minutes • **Serves 4**

If you're tired of the same old chicken, nothing amps up poultry like a tangy, mildly sweet glaze. You can easily replace the ponzu sauce with a clean-ingredient teriyaki or other Asian sauce. The initial sear on the chicken happens on the stovetop and then the dish finishes in the oven. So, relax and put your feet up before dinner.

¼ cup coconut oil, divided

1 pound boneless, skinless chicken breasts, cut into 1-inch pieces

¼ cup ponzu sauce (I like the Wan Ja Shu brand)

3 broccoli heads, chopped

½ teaspoon salt

2 tablespoons sesame seeds

Sriracha or red chili paste (optional)

Basil, for garnishing (optional)

1. Preheat the oven to 350°F.

2. In a large ovenproof dish or pot set over medium heat, heat 2 tablespoons of coconut oil. Add the chicken and sauté for 10 minutes. Stir in the ponzu sauce until well combined. Turn off the heat.

3. Add the broccoli and sprinkle with the salt.

4. Cover the pot and bake for 20 minutes. Remove the lid and cook for 5 minutes more.

5. Sprinkle with the sesame seeds and drizzle sriracha or garnish with basil (if using) and serve.

PREP TIP: If you don't have a pot that can transition from stovetop to oven, sear the chicken in a sauté pan first and then transfer it to an ovenproof dish before adding the broccoli.

Per Serving: Calories: 470; Total fat: 25g; Saturated fat: 13g; Sodium: 425mg; Carbohydrates: 28g; Fiber: 4g; Sugar: 20g; Protein: 38g

Baked Turkey Meatballs with Zucchini Noodles

Dairy-Free, Gluten-Free, No Added Sugar, Nut-Free, Soy-Free
Prep time: 15 minutes / **Cook time:** 25 minutes • **Serves** 4

This recipe calls for lean ground turkey, which is not quite as moist as the darker meat, so the meatballs hold together better. If you can't find lean turkey, add 1 to 2 additional tablespoons of chickpea, brown rice, or almond flour.

For the noodles

½ cup extra-virgin olive oil
½ cup fresh basil
2 garlic cloves (optional)
4 zucchini, spiralized or cut into long noodles with a peeler

For the meatballs

1 pound lean ground turkey
3 tablespoons chickpea flour
1 teaspoon salt
1 teaspoon freshly ground black pepper

To make the noodles

1. In a blender, blend together the olive oil, basil, and garlic (if using).

2. Add the mixture to a large bowl with the zucchini noodles and toss to coat.

To make the meatballs

3. Preheat the oven to 350°F. Line a baking sheet with parchment paper. In a medium bowl, mix the ground turkey, chickpea flour, salt, and pepper.

4. Using 1 tablespoon for each, roll the mixture into meatballs and place them on the prepared sheet. Bake for 20 to 25 minutes, or until lightly browned and cooked through.

5. Combine the meatballs with the zucchini noodles and serve.

Per Serving: Calories: 444; Total fat: 34g; Saturated fat: 6g; Sodium: 659mg; Carbohydrates: 12g; Fiber: 4g; Sugar: 4g; Protein: 27g

Garlic-Roasted Chicken with Celery

Gluten-Free, No Added Sugar, Nut-Free, Soy-Free
Prep time: 10 minutes / **Cook time:** 1 hour 15 minutes • **Serves** 4

This is a take on a classic French preparation for roast chicken. Cooking it in a Dutch oven keeps the chicken very moist. Make sure to use a high-quality olive oil for superior flavor and polyphenols; it should have a slight bitter or spicy aftertaste that "pinches" the throat.

1 (3½- to 4-pound) chicken, patted dry with paper towels

1 teaspoon salt

½ teaspoon black pepper

3 tablespoons extra-virgin olive oil

3 celery stalks, thinly sliced

2 shallots, thinly sliced

1 carrot, peeled and thinly sliced (optional)

4 garlic cloves

1 cup water

½ cup white wine

1. Preheat the oven to 400°F.

2. Season the chicken with the salt and pepper.

3. In a Dutch oven on the stove, warm the olive oil over medium heat. Place the chicken, breast-side down, in the pot, and brown the breast meat for 3 to 4 minutes. Remove from the pot and set aside.

4. Add the celery, shallots, carrot (if using), and garlic and sauté until softened, about 5 minutes.

5. Place the chicken, breast-side up, on top of the vegetables, and add the water and wine.

continued >>

6. Cover the pot, transfer to the oven, and roast the chicken until the juices at the thigh are no longer pink, about 1 hour. Remove from the oven and let rest for about 5 minutes before cutting into serving pieces.

7. Serve the chicken with the roasting vegetables and juices.

VARIATION TIP: Leftover chicken can be used in many other recipes in this book, such as a protein option in Stuffed Sweet Potatoes (page 60), Chickpea and Kale Salad (page 57), Sesame Chicken Stir-Fry (page 87), or Coconut Chicken Curry (page 88), allowing you to reduce cooking time. Store, covered, in the refrigerator for up to 5 days.

Per Serving: Calories: 527; Total fat: 35g; Saturated fat: 10g; Sodium: 685mg; Carbohydrates: 7g; Fiber: 1g; Sugar: 1g; Protein: 39g

Sesame Chicken Stir-Fry

Dairy-Free, Gluten-Free
Prep time: 15 minutes / **Cook time:** 25 minutes • **Serves 6**

Stir-fries are handy meals when you're short on time, ingredients, and patience. This stir-fry relies heavily on nutty sesame flavor, so it's for devoted sesame lovers. There is a double dose of calcium here from the tahini and the kale, making it a great option if you're looking to build or maintain bone health. As with all stir-fries, this one welcomes any extra vegetables in your refrigerator looking for a repurpose.

¾ cup warm water
½ cup tahini
¼ cup plus 2 tablespoons toasted sesame
    oil, divided
2 garlic cloves, minced
½ teaspoon salt

1 pound boneless, skinless chicken breasts,
    cut into ½-inch cubes
6 cups lightly packed kale, thoroughly
    washed and chopped
1 tablespoon tamari or coconut aminos
    (optional)

1. In a medium bowl, whisk together the warm water, tahini, ¼ cup of sesame oil, garlic, and salt.

2. In a large skillet on medium heat, heat the remaining 2 tablespoons of sesame oil.

3. Add the chicken and cook for 8 to 10 minutes, stirring occasionally. Stir in the tahini-sesame sauce, mixing well to coat the chicken. Cook for 6 to 8 minutes more.

4. One handful at a time, add the kale. When the first handful wilts, add the next. Continue until all the kale has been added. Drizzle tamari (if using) and serve hot.

VARIATION TIP: Boneless, skinless chicken thighs can also be used in this recipe.

Per Serving: Calories: 417; Total fat: 30g; Saturated fat: 3g; Sodium: 311mg; Carbohydrates: 12g; Fiber: 3g; Sugar: 0g; Protein: 27g

Coconut Chicken Curry

Dairy-Free, Gluten-Free, Soy-Free

Prep time: 8 minutes / **Cook time:** 35 minutes • **Serves 6**

This five-ingredient curry is quick, easy, and tasty. Most of the curry-like flavor stems from the curry powder, which you can adjust to suit your taste. Because curry mixes often contain chili powder, there's a chili-free alternative in the tip. This is also a great option for those who can't tolerate, or just dislike, spicy food. This recipe is higher in saturated fat, so pair it with lower-fat meals for the rest of the day if you are sensitive to saturated-fat intake. I love to provide a toppings buffet for people to customize their bowls—try chopped cilantro, sliced serrano peppers, lime wedges, and cayenne pepper.

3 cups canned coconut milk

2 cups water

3 tablespoons curry powder

1 tablespoon garam masala (optional)

2 pounds boneless, skinless chicken thighs, cut into cubes

1 white onion, chopped

1 teaspoon salt

3 bunches Swiss chard, washed, stemmed, and coarsely chopped

1 (15-ounce) can chickpeas, drained and rinsed (optional)

1. In a large saucepan, combine the coconut milk, water, curry powder, garam masala (if using), chicken, onion, and salt. Bring to a boil over high heat, reduce the heat to low, cover, and simmer for 30 minutes.

2. Add the Swiss chard and chickpeas (if using) to the saucepan. Cook for 5 minutes, or until the chard wilts and the chickpeas are warm.

VARIATION TIP: To make this without nightshades, make your own quick, chile-free version of curry powder. In a small bowl, whisk together 2 teaspoons of ground cumin, 1 teaspoon of ground coriander, 1 teaspoon of ground ginger, and ½ teaspoon of ground turmeric. Add the spices to the curry, taste, and adjust as needed.

Per Serving (without chickpeas): Calories: 581; Total fat: 40g; Saturated fat: 21g; Sodium: 552mg; Carbohydrates: 10g; Fiber: 4g; Sugar: 5g; Protein: 48g

Walnut-Crusted Salmon Fillets

Dairy-Free, Gluten-Free, Omega-3-Rich, Soy-Free
Prep time: 10 minutes / **Cook time:** 20 minutes • **Serves 4**

Omega-3 fats are the ultimate anti-inflammatory nutrients and are required in the human diet because our bodies cannot make them. EPA and DHA are animal-based omega-3s (rich in salmon) and are absorbed well, while ALA (rich in walnuts) is the plant-based omega-3, which is not as well-absorbed but still beneficial. This walnut and salmon combination tops the omega-3 charts and is a delicious spin on a traditional bread crumb coating.

1 tablespoon extra-virgin olive oil, divided

1 pound skin-on salmon fillet

½ cup walnuts, finely chopped

6 chive stalks, minced

1 teaspoon sea salt

1 teaspoon dried dill

1 tablespoon freshly squeezed lemon juice

1. Preheat the oven to 350°F and line a baking sheet with parchment paper or foil.

2. Brush half of the oil on all sides of the salmon and place skin-side down on the prepared baking sheet.

3. In a small bowl, mix the walnuts, chives, salt, and dill. Stir in the lemon juice and the remaining ½ tablespoon olive oil. Gently press the mixture onto the top side of the salmon fillet.

4. Bake for 10 to 12 minutes or until the salmon is cooked through and flakes easily. Carefully transfer the salmon to plates, to keep the topping in place.

VARIATION TIP: Substitute pistachios for the walnuts for a buttery, piney flavor. Or, to make this nut-free, replace the walnuts with chopped pumpkin seeds.

Per Serving: Calories: 262; Total fat: 17g; Saturated fat: 3g; Sodium: 410mg; Carbohydrates: 2g; Fiber: 1g; Sugar: 0g; Protein: 26g

Mediterranean Mackerel

Dairy-Free, Gluten-Free, Omega-3-Rich, Soy-Free
Prep time: 10 minutes / **Cook time:** 20 minutes • **Serves** 4

Jazz up canned fish in no time with this recipe. Choose Atlantic mackerel or Atka mackerel for high omega-3s and low mercury. I love the BELA or King Oscar brands. If the mackerel is in tomato sauce, don't drain the cans. Add all components to the casserole dish for more flavor and nutrition. You can replace the canned mackerel with 1 pound of fresh fish if you prefer. I like to serve this recipe over a bed of arugula or spinach, with additional vegetables for a low-carb meal, or with Pesto Lentil Pasta (page 62) for a full spread.

4 (4-ounce) cans mackerel fillets, drained

1½ cups cherry tomatoes

2 tablespoons dry white wine

8 garlic-stuffed olives, halved (optional)

Grated zest and juice of 1 lemon

Freshly ground black pepper

Salt

6 thyme or oregano sprigs (optional)

4 cups arugula (optional)

1. Preheat the oven to 350°F.

2. In a casserole dish, arrange the fillets. Add the tomatoes, white wine, and olives (if using) on the top and sides. Sprinkle with lemon zest and juice, pepper, salt, and fresh herbs (if using).

3. Bake for 18 to 20 minutes or until the cherry tomatoes have burst and the fish is starting to crisp up on the edges. Serve over a bed of 1 cup arugula (if desired).

Per Serving: Calories: 145; Total fat: 6g; Saturated fat: 2g; Sodium: 364mg; Carbohydrates: 3g; Fiber: 1g; Sugar: 2g; Protein: 20g

Salt and Vinegar Anchovy Potato Salad

Dairy-Free, Gluten-Free, Omega-3-Rich, Soy-Free
Prep time: 15 minutes, plus 30 minutes to chill / **Cook time:** 20 minutes • **Serves** 4

This is my simplified, healthier take on German potato salad. Enjoy omega-3s from the anchovies, as well as potassium from the potatoes. Potato skins are rich in nutrients, so don't peel them. Potassium is an essential nutrient for healthy heart function and fluid balance, helps offset sodium's effects, and is especially important for those taking corticosteroid medications.

1 pound red potatoes, quartered
1 (4-ounce) can anchovies in olive oil, coarsely chopped
⅓ small red onion, diced, divided
¼ cup packed parsley, chopped, divided

1 teaspoon salt
¼ teaspoon freshly ground black pepper
⅓ cup red wine vinegar
3 tablespoons extra-virgin olive oil

1. Fill a large pot with a steamer insert with about 1 inch of water and bring to a boil over high heat. Add the potatoes and steam for 20 minutes or until fork-tender.

2. Transfer the potatoes to a medium bowl and lightly mash, then add the anchovies, half the onion, half the parsley, the salt, and the pepper, and stir.

3. In a blender, pulse the remaining half onion, remaining 2 tablespoons parsley, the vinegar, and the oil for about 1 minute until emulsified. Pour the mixture over the potatoes and stir. Taste and season with more salt, pepper, or vinegar as desired. Chill for at least 30 minutes before serving.

PREP TIP: Steam the potatoes ahead of time and refrigerate for up to 3 days. Cooking, then cooling the potatoes helps some of the starch convert into resistant starch, which is a type of carbohydrate that isn't absorbed; it feeds your gut bacteria.

Per Serving (1 cup): Calories: 221; Total fat: 12g; Saturated fat: 2g; Sodium: 1,076mg; Carbohydrates: 19g; Fiber: 2g; Sugar: 2g; Protein: 8g

Baked Salmon Patties with Greens

Dairy-Free, Gluten-Free, No Added Sugar, Omega-3-Rich, Soy-Free
Prep time: 15 minutes / **Cook time:** 35 To 38 minutes • **Serves 4**

My siblings and I grew up eating whatever animals my dad hunted or fished himself—deer, quail, duck, and a wide variety of fish—so I've always enjoyed seafood. Whether you've loved fish all your life or are just venturing into eating seafood, fish cakes are a great solution for increasing omega-3 intake. While I prefer and recommend using canned salmon with bones to increase calcium intake, you can use boneless canned salmon if you find the soft bones unpalatable.

2 cups cooked, mashed sweet potatoes
  (about 2 large sweet potatoes)
2 (6-ounce) cans wild salmon, drained
¼ cup almond flour
¼ teaspoon ground turmeric

2 tablespoons olive oil
2 kale bunches, thoroughly washed,
  stemmed, and cut into ribbons
¼ teaspoon salt

1. Preheat the oven to 350°F. Line a baking sheet with parchment paper.

2. In a large bowl, stir together the mashed sweet potatoes, salmon, almond flour, and turmeric.

3. Using a ⅓-cup measure, scoop the salmon mixture onto the prepared baking sheet. Flatten slightly with the bottom of the measuring cup. Repeat with the remaining mixture. Bake for 30 minutes, flipping the patties halfway through.

4. In a large skillet set over medium heat, heat the oil. Add the kale and sauté for 5 to 8 minutes, or until the kale is bright and wilted. Sprinkle with the salt and serve with the salmon patties.

VARIATION TIP: To make this recipe nut-free, in a spice grinder or blender, grind 3 tablespoons of sunflower or pumpkin seeds to a fine meal.

Per Serving: Calories: 320; Total fat: 13g; Saturated fat: 1g; Sodium: 88mg; Carbohydrates: 32g; Fiber: 5g; Sugar: 0g; Protein: 21g

Lemony Salmon with Mixed Vegetables

Dairy-Free, Gluten-Free, No Added Sugar, Nut-Free, Omega-3-Rich, Soy-Free
Prep time: 10 minutes / **Cook time:** 15 to 20 minutes • **Serves** 4

The pairing of wild salmon and lemon is fresh and appealing. Aside from its delicious taste, the salmon's anti-inflammatory omega-3 fats will help you better absorb the nutrients in the vegetables—particularly the vitamin C and antioxidants. How's that for a power couple? Replace the individual vegetables with a fresh or frozen bag of California blend vegetables to minimize prep.

4 (5-ounce) wild salmon fillets

1 teaspoon salt, divided

1 teaspoon black pepper, divided

2 lemons, 1 washed and sliced thin and
  1 quartered

1 broccoli head, coarsely chopped

1 cauliflower head, coarsely chopped

1 small bunch (4 to 6) carrots, cut into coins

1 tablespoon fresh herbs such as thyme
  and chopped parsley (optional)

1. Preheat the oven to 400°F. Line a baking sheet with parchment paper.

2. Place the salmon on the prepared sheet and sprinkle with ½ teaspoon each of salt and pepper. Drape each fillet with a few lemon slices.

3. Bake for 15 minutes, or until the salmon is opaque and flakes easily with a fork.

4. While the salmon cooks, fill a saucepan with 3 inches of water and insert a steamer basket. Bring to a boil over high heat. Add the broccoli, cauliflower, and carrots to the saucepan. Cover and steam for 6 to 8 minutes, or until they are fork-tender. Sprinkle with the remaining ½ teaspoon of salt and pepper.

continued >>

5. Top each salmon fillet with a heaping pile of vegetables, a sprinkle of fresh herbs (if using), a squeeze of fresh lemon, and serve.

PREP TIP: Replace the whole vegetables with a 24-ounce bag of California blend vegetables, either fresh or frozen, to cut down on prep time. Follow the cooking directions, sprinkle with salt and pepper, then proceed to step 5.

VARIATION TIP: Broccoli, cauliflower, and carrots create a simple, inexpensive side dish, but you can use any of your favorite vegetables to complement the salmon. Summer squash works well, or any variety of fresh or steamed hardy leafy greens.

Per Serving: Calories: 330; Total fat: 13g; Saturated fat: 2g; Sodium: 761mg; Carbohydrates: 20g; Fiber: 7g; Sugar: 8g; Protein: 35g

Spiced Trout and Spinach

Dairy-Free, Gluten-Free, No Added Sugar, Nut-Free, Omega-3-Rich, Soy-Free
Prep time: 10 minutes / **Cook time:** 15 minutes • **Serves** 4

Trout is typically available year-round. It's a freshwater fish, and even people who claim they don't like fish often enjoy it. In addition, the Environmental Working Group reports that farmed or freshwater small trout—such as rainbow trout—are low in mercury and other contaminants such as polychlorinated biphenyls (PCBs) yet high in omega-3 fats. These characteristics do not apply to the larger-bodied trout species known as sea trout, saltwater trout, and lake trout. This trout is baked on a bed of spinach for a low-carb, nutrient-dense meal. To add complex carbs for a balanced meal, pair it with Chipotle Sweet Potato and Cauliflower Soup (page 48) or Garlic-Lime Black Beans (page 41).

Extra-virgin olive oil, for brushing
½ red onion, thinly sliced
1 (10-ounce) package frozen spinach, thawed
4 boneless freshwater trout fillets

1 teaspoon salt
¼ teaspoon chipotle powder (optional)
¼ teaspoon garlic powder
2 tablespoons freshly squeezed lemon juice

1. Preheat the oven to 375°F. Brush a 9-by-13-inch baking pan with olive oil.

2. Scatter the red onion and spinach in the pan and lay the trout fillets on the spinach.

3. Sprinkle the fish with salt, chipotle powder (if using), and garlic powder, cover with aluminum foil, and bake until the trout is firm, about 15 minutes.

4. Drizzle with the lemon juice and serve.

VARIATION TIP: Another mild whitefish, such as cod, halibut, or pollock, would also work well in this dish. Stronger-tasting fish will permeate the spinach, compromising its natural flavor.

Per Serving: Calories: 160; Total fat: 7g; Saturated fat: 1g; Sodium: 670mg; Carbohydrates: 5g; Fiber: 2g; Sugar: 1g; Protein: 19g

Basic Baked Salmon

Dairy-Free, Gluten-Free, Nut-Free, Omega-3-Rich, Soy-Free
Prep time: 5 minutes / **Cook time:** 15 minutes • **Serves 4**

The moistness of salmon makes it an excellent fish for almost any preparation. This version is simply prepared with salt, pepper, and lemon juice, then baked. Be sure to let it rest for 5 to 10 minutes after taking it out of the oven because it will continue to gently cook. If you want to meal prep, double the recipe and eat the other half for lunch over a simple bed of fresh baby spinach for a quick salad.

Extra-virgin olive oil, for brushing the pan

4 (3- to 4-ounce) boneless salmon fillets

1 teaspoon salt

¼ teaspoon freshly ground black pepper

2 tablespoons freshly squeezed lemon juice

1. Preheat the oven to 375°F. Lightly brush a 9-inch square baking pan with oil.

2. Place the salmon in the pan, skin-side down (if it has skin). Season with salt and pepper, then drizzle with the lemon juice.

3. Bake until the fish is cooked through and flaky, 10 to 15 minutes.

4. Remove from the oven and let rest for 5 to 10 minutes. Using a spatula, gently lift the salmon off the baked skin before serving.

PREP TIP: Not sure if the salmon is done? There are two ways to tell. You can touch the salmon at the thickest part and see if it's firm—if it is, then it's done. You can also use a fork to gently pull apart one or two of the flakes of the fillets in the thickest part. If it's still bright pink inside, return it to the oven for a few more minutes.

Per Serving: Calories: 180; Total fat: 11g; Saturated fat: 1g; Sodium: 630mg; Carbohydrates: 0g; Fiber: 0g; Sugar: 0g; Protein: 19g

Sardine Donburi

Dairy-Free, Gluten-Free, Nut-Free, Omega-3-Rich
Prep time: 10 minutes / **Cook time:** 45 to 50 minutes • **Serves 4**

Sardine Donburi is a Japanese dish that my kids say tastes like deconstructed sushi. Sardines get a bad rap, but they shouldn't. Sardines are an amazing source of low-mercury, anti-inflammatory omega-3 fats, protein, and bone-building vitamin D and calcium. Replace the olive oil with sesame oil and add a drizzle of soy sauce or tamari to each bowl for a more authentic flavor.

1½ cups brown rice, rinsed well

3 cups water

½ teaspoon salt

3 (4-ounce) cans sardines packed in olive oil, oil reserved

3 scallions, white and green parts, sliced thin

1-inch piece fresh ginger, peeled and grated

2 teaspoons rice vinegar

Sriracha for serving (optional)

1. In a large saucepan, combine the rice, water, and salt. Bring to a boil over high heat, reduce the heat to low, cover, and simmer for 45 to 50 minutes, or until tender.

2. In a medium bowl, mash the sardines.

3. When the rice is done, add the sardines, scallions, and ginger to the saucepan. Mix thoroughly.

4. Divide the rice among four bowls. Drizzle each bowl with 1 teaspoon of the reserved oil, ½ teaspoon of rice vinegar, and sriracha (if using).

PREP TIP: Don't have the time to wait for brown rice to cook? Use a pressure cooker to cut the cook time by half. Or use quinoa or buckwheat instead, as these will cook in 15 to 20 minutes. Leftover rice is great, too; just rewarm it in a skillet on the stove.

Per Serving (1⅓ cup): Calories: 640; Total fat: 24g; Saturated fat: 1g; Sodium: 499mg; Carbohydrates: 74g; Fiber: 4g; Sugar: 0g; Protein: 25g

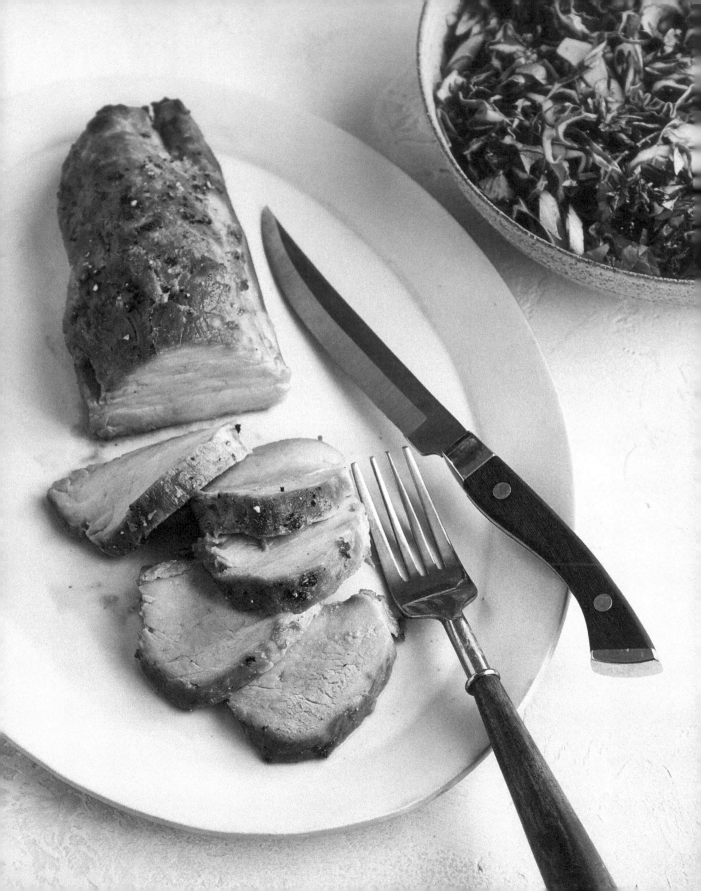

CHAPTER 7

PORK, BEEF, AND LAMB

Pork Verde Tacos

Dairy-Free, Gluten-Free, Nut-Free, Soy-Free

Prep time: 10 minutes / **Cook time:** 35 minutes • **Serves 4**

Tacos are a family favorite in my house, and I love how customizable they are. Pick a protein and sauce, create a buffet of toppings, and—voilà!—everyone is happy. Replace tortillas with Swiss chard or cabbage leaves to up your cruciferous veggie intake or try Savory Lentil Flatbread (page 38) as your tortilla alternative. I recommend serving this with Garlic-Lime Black Beans (page 41) for a bump in fiber and complex carbohydrates.

1 teaspoon salt

½ teaspoon black pepper

1 teaspoon ground cumin

1 pound pork tenderloin

1 tablespoon olive oil

1 (16-ounce) jar tomatillo (green) salsa, divided

8 (6-inch) grain-free or corn tortillas (I love the El Milagro and Siete brands)

½ cup fresh prepared guacamole

1 cup fresh spinach, chopped (optional)

½ bunch cilantro, chopped (optional)

1 jalapeño pepper, chopped (optional)

1. Preheat the oven to 325°F.

2. Sprinkle the salt, pepper, and cumin on all sides of the pork.

3. In an ovenproof medium pot with a lid (or a Dutch oven), heat the oil over medium-high heat. Add the pork and sear it on all sides.

4. Add the salsa (reserve ¼ cup for topping) and stir to coat the pork evenly. Bring back to a simmer, then cover, transfer whole pot to the oven and cook for 30 to 35 minutes.

5. Slice or shred, and serve warm in tortillas topped with 1 tablespoon guacamole, 1 tablespoon salsa, spinach (if using), cilantro (if using), and jalapeño pepper (if using).

VARIATION TIP: If you're looking to speed up the cooking process, season the pork tenderloin with salt, pepper, and cumin, then sear it on all sides in 1 tablespoon of oil in a pressure cooker. Add 12 ounces of salsa, then mix to make sure there is salsa and moisture under the pork. Cook on high pressure for 20 minutes, then natural release for 5 minutes. If batch cooking, for every extra pound of pork above 1 pound, add 20 more minutes. Carefully open the lid and shred with two forks. Serve as directed above.

Per Serving (2 tacos): Calories: 363; Total fat: 13g; Saturated fat: 3g; Sodium: 978mg; Carbohydrates: 35g; Fiber: 7g; Sugar: 5g; Protein: 29g

Pork Tenderloin with Warm Tomato Dressing

Dairy-Free, Gluten-Free, Nut-Free, Soy-Free
Prep time: 15 minutes / **Cook time:** 20 minutes • **Serves** 4

This tangy tomato dressing is a client and family favorite and can be spooned over proteins, vegetables, and/or whole grains. I love pairing this recipe with Warm Garlic Greens (page 55) or Chickpea and Kale Salad (page 57).

3 garlic cloves

1 pound pork tenderloin

4 teaspoons extra-virgin olive oil, divided

1¼ teaspoons salt, divided

½ teaspoon freshly ground black pepper

1 pint (10 ounces) cherry tomatoes

⅔ cup dry red wine

¼ cup balsamic vinegar

1 tablespoon sugar (optional)

1 teaspoon red-wine vinegar (optional)

1. Preheat the oven to 400°F. Mince the garlic and let rest for 10 minutes.

2. Brush the tenderloin with 1 teaspoon of olive oil and season with 1 teaspoon of salt and the pepper.

3. Heat an ovenproof skillet over medium-high heat, add 1 teaspoon of oil and sear the pork on all sides, 3 to 4 minutes total. Roast for about 15 minutes or until the pork reaches the internal temperature of 145°F.

4. In a medium saucepan over medium heat on the stove, cook the remaining 2 teaspoons olive oil and the tomatoes, stirring often, until the tomatoes are blistered, about 5 minutes. Stir in the red wine, balsamic vinegar, and garlic, and cook for about 5 minutes, or until the liquid is reduced by half. Add the remaining ¼ teaspoon of salt, the sugar (if using), and the red wine vinegar (if using), and cook for about 1 more minute.

5. Let the sauce cool slightly and spoon over the tenderloin before serving.

Per Serving: Calories: 233; Total fat: 8g; Saturated fat: 2g; Sodium: 648mg; Carbohydrates: 6g; Fiber: 1g; Sugar: 4g; Protein: 24g

Banh Mi Pork

Dairy-Free, Gluten-Free, Nut-Free
Prep time: 15 minutes, plus 30 minutes to 1 day to chill / **Cook time:** 10 minutes
Serves 6

Banh mi is a flavorful Vietnamese dish of seasoned pork topped with pickled vegetables, such as radishes, carrots, cucumbers, and jalapeños. This recipe enables you to make the pork base, so you can load it up with your preference of pickled toppings. My personal twist is to add sauerkraut on top of the other marinated vegetables for a boost in probiotics. Serve the banh mi pork in a bowl by itself topped with vegetables, in lettuce wraps, or on toasted sourdough buns (if eating gluten) smeared with mayonnaise.

2 tablespoons fish sauce

1 tablespoon extra-virgin olive oil, divided

1 tablespoon rice vinegar

1 tablespoon honey

2 garlic cloves, minced

1 teaspoon salt

½ teaspoon black pepper

1 pound pork tenderloin, thinly sliced

2 cups pickled vegetables, divided
  (optional; see Tip)

¼ cup sauerkraut, divided (optional)

¼ cup chopped cilantro, divided (optional)

Sriracha (optional)

1. In a medium glass bowl, mix the fish sauce, oil, vinegar, honey, garlic, salt, and pepper. Stir in the pork, cover, and chill for 30 minutes up to 1 day. Thread the pork onto skewers. Meanwhile, mince the garlic and set aside at least 10 minutes.

2. Heat an indoor or outdoor grill to medium-high heat. Place the skewers on the grill, brush with the remaining marinade, and close the lid. Grill for about 8 minutes in total, turning once or twice to prevent burning and ensure even cooking. Cool slightly.

continued >>

3. Divide the pork among the bowls. Top with pickled vegetables (if using), and optional toppings of choice.

PREP TIP: To make pickled vegetables, in a small saucepan over medium heat, heat a mixture of ½ cup rice vinegar, ¼ cup water, ¼ teaspoon salt, and 1 tablespoon sugar of your choice and stir until dissolved, about 3 minutes. Let cool. Fill a 16-ounce jar with 2 cups of your choice of matchstick carrots, daikon radishes (or use red radishes), cucumbers, and jalapeños (if desired). Pour the cooled liquid over top. Add equal parts of vinegar and water until the liquid covers all vegetables in the jar. Cover and refrigerate for at least 1 hour and enjoy within 1 week.

VARIATION TIP: To skip the grill, place the skewers in a casserole dish and roast in a 400°F oven for 10 to 12 minutes.

Per Serving: Calories: 125; Total fat: 5g; Saturated fat: 1g; Sodium: 793mg; Carbohydrates: 3g; Fiber: 0g; Sugar: 3g; Protein: 16g

Smoky Coppa and Collard Greens

Dairy-Free, Gluten-Free, No Added Sugar, Nut-Free, Soy-Free
Prep time: 15 minutes / **Cook time:** 55 minutes • **Serves 6** (½ cup)

This recipe is my family's favorite way to eat dark leafy greens (kids included!). Small servings of cured meats can be enjoyed as flavoring for nutrient-dense greens. Coppa, also known as capicola or cappocola, is an Italian dry-aged meat made from pork shoulder and is like a cross between sausage and prosciutto. It often has a seasoned coating and is rich in protein, vitamin B_{12}, and flavor.

2 garlic cloves

4 ounces coppa, chopped (see Tip)

1 tablespoon extra-virgin olive oil

16 ounces chopped collard greens (about 12 cups)

2 cups water

2 large leeks, both white and green parts, sliced

¼ cup red wine vinegar

1 teaspoon salt

Hot sauce, for serving (optional)

1. Mince the garlic and set aside for 10 minutes. In a large saucepan with a lid over medium heat, add the coppa and cook until crispy, about 5 minutes.

2. Add the olive oil and garlic and sauté for 2 to 3 minutes.

3. Stir in the collards, water, leeks, vinegar, and salt. Cover and simmer for 40 to 45 minutes until the greens and leeks have softened. Serve with hot sauce (if using), or more salt and vinegar if desired.

VARIATION TIP: You can replace the coppa with a smoked turkey leg, ham hock, bacon, or another cured pork, but the taste and total fat in the dish will vary.

Per Serving: Calories: 137; Total fat: 9g; Saturated fat: 3g; Sodium: 689mg; Carbohydrates: 9g; Fiber: 4g; Sugar: 2g; Protein: 8g

Sausage and Cabbage Skillet

Dairy-Free, Gluten-Free, Nut-Free, Soy-Free
Prep time: 15 minutes / **Cook time:** 25 minutes • **4 to 6 servings**

Cabbage is in the cruciferous family, and this recipe emphasizes a higher volume of cabbage versus sausage as a delicious way to reap the cabbage's benefits. My husband and I like to drizzle Tabasco or add cayenne pepper to our plates while my kids enjoy the milder version.

4 garlic cloves, divided

1 tablespoon plus 1 teaspoon extra-virgin olive oil, divided

12 ounces smoked 100% grass-fed beef sausage, sliced

1 yellow onion, diced

1 large head green cabbage, cored and coarsely chopped

2 large carrots, peeled and chopped

1 teaspoon salt

½ teaspoon freshly ground black pepper

1 tablespoon red wine vinegar (optional)

1. Mince the garlic and set aside for 10 minutes. Heat 1 teaspoon of oil in a large skillet with a lid over medium-high heat. Stir in the sausage and cook until browned, 3 to 5 minutes. Transfer the sausage (keeping the drippings) from the skillet onto a paper-towel-lined plate.

2. Reduce the heat to medium-low, add the remaining 1 tablespoon of oil, and sauté the onion for 2 to 3 minutes or until softened. Add half of the garlic and sauté for another 1 to 2 minutes.

3. Stir in the cabbage, carrots, salt, and pepper. Cover and cook about 10 minutes until the cabbage and carrots have softened. Uncover and add the remaining garlic and red wine vinegar (if using). Cook for another 2 to 3 minutes.

4. Serve hot and season with more salt or pepper to taste.

Per Serving: Calories: 332; Total fat: 17g; Saturated fat: 5g; Sodium: 921mg; Carbohydrates: 32g; Fiber: 9g; Sugar: 15g; Protein: 16g

Sheet Pan Sausage, Pear, and Brussels Sprouts

Dairy-Free, Gluten-Free, No Added Sugar, Nut-Free, Soy-Free
Prep time: 10 minutes / **Cook time:** 35 minutes • **Serves** 4

Sheet pan dinners are some of my favorite meals for the family. Load up the pan with a variety of ingredients, bake while you multitask, and enjoy a healthy meal with speedy cleanup. Substitutions are easy for this recipe; replace the bratwurst with chicken sausage, boneless pork chops, or chicken thighs if you prefer. Add sliced sweet potatoes or winter squash for another layer of flavor and nutrition.

1 pound Brussels sprouts, trimmed and halved

3 shallots, quartered

2 firm-ripe pears, cored, cut into wedges

6 thyme sprigs

1 tablespoon extra-virgin olive oil

½ teaspoon salt

½ teaspoon freshly ground black pepper

1 pound bratwurst, or 4 links

¼ cup sauerkraut (optional)

Dijon or spicy brown mustard for serving (optional)

1. Preheat the oven to 400°F. Line a baking sheet with parchment paper.

2. Spread the Brussels sprouts, shallots, pears, thyme, and oil on the prepared baking sheet, using your hands to evenly coat everything. Sprinkle with salt and pepper and mix again. Arrange the bratwurst on top of the vegetables.

3. Bake for 25 to 30 minutes. Remove the baking sheet from the oven, distribute the sauerkraut on the vegetables (if using) and mix lightly. Serve warm with mustard (if using).

Per Serving: Calories: 418; Total fat: 29g; Saturated fat: 9g; Sodium: 899mg; Carbohydrates: 27g; Fiber: 7g; Sugar: 12g; Protein: 16g

Spinach and Sweet Potato Bacon Hash

Dairy-Free, Gluten-Free, No Added Sugar, Nut-Free, Soy-Free

Prep time: 10 minutes / **Cook time:** 20 minutes • **Serves** 4

While I don't recommend bacon as a daily staple, when used intentionally and in small amounts, bacon can provide rich flavor to other nutrient-dense ingredients. In addition, this recipe discards the bacon grease, helping reduce the saturated fat content. When nutritious food tastes good, you're apt to cook it—and eat it—more frequently. I love topping this hash with poached or fried eggs.

6 bacon slices

1 (10-ounce) package frozen chopped spinach

¼ cup water

2 medium sweet potatoes, cubed

1 small red onion, chopped

2 tablespoons extra-virgin olive oil

½ teaspoon salt

¼ teaspoon freshly ground black pepper

½ cup sauerkraut (optional)

Hot sauce for serving (optional)

1. Heat a large ovenproof skillet over medium-high heat. Put in the bacon, cook for about 3 minutes, flip, and cook for another 3 minutes, or until mostly crispy. Transfer the bacon to a plate, discard the grease, and lightly wipe out the skillet with a paper towel.

2. Return the skillet to medium-high heat and put in the spinach and water. Cook until the moisture is absorbed and the spinach is thawed/warmed, about 5 minutes. Transfer the spinach to one side of the plate with the bacon.

3. Put the sweet potato, onion, and oil in the empty skillet, stir, cover, and cook for 10 minutes, stirring occasionally. Uncover, stir, and cook until the potatoes are tender, 5 to 10 more minutes. Add the spinach, bacon, salt, and pepper. Stir and cook until all components are heated through. Serve hot, topped with the sauerkraut (if using) and a drizzle of hot sauce (if using).

Per Serving: Calories: 224; Total fat: 13g; Saturated fat: 3g; Sodium: 670mg; Carbohydrates: 18g; Fiber: 4g; Sugar: 4g; Protein: 10g

Simple Pan-Seared Pork Loin

Dairy-Free, Gluten-Free, No Added Sugar, Nut-Free, Soy-Free
Prep time: 15 minutes / **Cook time:** 35 minutes • **Serves** 8

Pork offers a nice break from chicken and seafood. Though this juicy meat lags behind quality chicken and beef when it comes to sustainable farming—which protects the land, people, communities, and animal welfare—pork farmers are catching up. Buying pork from the farmers' market is one way to ensure you're getting sustainably raised pork. This recipe pairs well with Sheet Pan Winter Vegetable Bake (page 63) or Tahini Kale Noodles (page 73).

1 cup water

1 (3-pound) boneless pork loin roast

2 tablespoons extra-virgin olive oil

1½ teaspoons salt

1 teaspoon dried rosemary, or 1 tablespoon fresh finely minced

½ teaspoon freshly ground black pepper

1. Preheat the oven to 375°F. Pour the water into a 9-by-13-inch roasting pan.

2. Heat a large skillet over high heat. Coat the roast with the olive oil and place it in the hot skillet. Brown on all sides, 2 to 3 minutes per side.

3. Transfer the browned roast to the roasting pan. Combine the salt, rosemary, and pepper in a small bowl and sprinkle the seasonings evenly over the meat.

4. Roast until a meat thermometer inserted in the center reads 150°F, 30 to 35 minutes.

5. Let the roast rest for about 10 minutes before cutting and serving.

PREP TIP: Searing the meat before roasting adds nice color and extra flavor to the roast while keeping the interior moist. You can use this same technique with beef or lamb.

Per Serving (4½ ounces): Calories: 242; Total fat: 14g; Saturated fat: 3g; Sodium: 496mg; Carbohydrates: 0g; Fiber: 0g; Sugar: 0g; Protein: 27g

Garlic Beef and Broccoli Stir-Fry

Dairy-Free, Gluten-Free, No Added Sugar, Nut-Free
Prep time: 15 minutes / **Cook time:** 20 minutes • **Serves 4**

Here, I choose flank steak, which is leaner than skirt steak but still has a robust flavor and doesn't require a marinade to be tender. Cooking leaner cuts of beef with moist heat helps keep the dish lower in saturated fat and calories. With antioxidant- and polyphenol-rich broccoli and ginger, you have yourself a dinner winner.

5 garlic cloves

2 medium heads broccoli, chopped

1 tablespoon extra-virgin olive oil

3 tablespoons tamari, plus more for serving

1 pound flank steak, thinly sliced

1 (1-inch) piece ginger, peeled and minced

½ teaspoon freshly ground black pepper

2 scallions, green and white parts, sliced, for serving (optional)

1 tablespoon sesame seeds, for serving (optional)

Sriracha, for serving (optional)

1. Mince the garlic and set aside for 10 minutes. Meanwhile, in a medium saucepan with a steamer insert, bring 1 inch of water to a simmer over medium-high heat. Add the broccoli and cover to steam until bright green and al dente, about 5 minutes. (It will continue to cook when it's added to the dish later.)

2. Heat a large skillet over medium-high heat and add the oil and tamari. Cook for 2 to 3 minutes until bubbly and reduced a bit. Add the beef and sauté until nearly done, about 5 minutes.

3. Add the garlic, ginger, steamed broccoli, and pepper. Cook for 2 to 3 minutes until the garlic is softened and aromatic and the beef is cooked through.

4. Taste and add more tamari, pepper, or salt as desired. Serve hot and sprinkle with scallions (if using), sesame seeds (if using), or sriracha (if using).

Per Serving: Calories: 344; Total fat: 14g; Saturated fat: 4g; Sodium: 917mg; Carbohydrates: 24g; Fiber: 8g; Sugar: 7g; Protein: 34g

Mushroom Beef Flax Meatballs

Dairy-Free, Gluten-Free, Nut-Free, Omega-3-Rich, Soy-Free
Prep time: 15 minutes / **Cook time:** 15 minutes • **4 to 6 servings**

Grass-fed cows eat their natural diet, which results in their meat containing higher levels of a healthy type of polyunsaturated fat—conjugated linoleic acid, or CLA. CLA helps reduce body fat by lowering inflammation, converting white fat to brown fat, and more. I love to pair these meatballs with cauliflower mashed potatoes, pea/lentil pasta with tomato sauce, or Tahini Kale Noodles (page 73).

1 pound 90% lean grass-fed ground beef or ground sirloin

3 ounces mushrooms, minced

3 tablespoons garlic marinara

1 tablespoon ground flaxseed

1 tablespoon Italian seasoning

1 tablespoon nutritional yeast (optional)

½ teaspoon salt

¼ teaspoon freshly ground black pepper

1. Preheat the oven to 400°F. Line a baking sheet with parchment paper.

2. In a medium bowl, combine the ground beef, mushrooms, marinara, flaxseed, Italian seasoning, nutritional yeast (if using), salt, and pepper, and mix with your hands until just combined.

3. Scoop a heaping tablespoon of meat in the palm of your hands and roll into a ball. Place on the prepared baking sheet and repeat until all the meat mixture is used, making about 20 meatballs.

4. Brush each meatball with olive oil and bake for 15 minutes. Cool slightly before serving.

VARIATION TIP: You can replace the 90% ground beef with lean or extra-lean ground turkey to reduce total fat, though the CLA content will be lower as well.

Per Serving: Calories: 216; Total fat: 12g; Saturated fat: 4g; Sodium: 368mg; Carbohydrates: 2g; Fiber: 1g; Sugar: 1g; Protein: 24g

Fajita Beef and Cilantro Cauliflower Bowl

Dairy-Free, Gluten-Free, No Added Sugar, Nut-Free, Soy-Free
Prep time: 15 minutes, plus 30 minutes to marinate / **Cook time:** 20 minutes • **Serves** 4

Seasoning mixes often contain preservatives or additives that may be triggering or inflammatory for some, so be careful what you choose. I love the Siete and Thrive Market brands for taco or fajita seasoning. This recipe serves a flavorful protein with a cilantro-flavored cauliflower for a boost of the health-promoting, sulfur-containing compounds glucosinolates. These phytochemicals are especially important to combine with meats that have been cooked at high temperatures that accrue carcinogens (though this recipe does not cook the beef that high).

1 pound flank steak, thinly sliced

1 tablespoon plus 2 teaspoons extra-virgin olive oil, divided

1½ tablespoons taco or fajita beef seasoning

Juice of 3 limes, divided

2 garlic cloves (optional)

16 ounces cauliflower rice, fresh or frozen

1 bunch cilantro, chopped

2 scallions, white and green parts, sliced (optional)

½ teaspoon salt

1 avocado (optional)

1. In a glass or nonreactive medium-size bowl, stir the steak, 2 teaspoons oil, the seasoning, and the juice of 1 lime to combine. Cover and refrigerate to marinate for at least 30 minutes. Mince the garlic and set aside for 10 minutes (if using).

2. During the last 10 minutes of marinating time, remove the meat from the refrigerator to allow it to come closer to room temperature. Meanwhile, cook the cauliflower.

3. In the same skillet over medium-high heat, cook 2 teaspoons of olive oil and the garlic (if using) for 1 to 2 minutes, until aromatic. Reduce the heat to medium and add the cauliflower rice. Stir, cover, and cook 3 to 4 minutes until the cauliflower has softened somewhat. (It will continue to cook.) Uncover, cook for an additional 1 to 2 minutes to cook off the extra moisture (or double the time for frozen rice), and allow the cauliflower to crisp up slightly.

4. Remove from the heat and stir in the cilantro, the remaining 2 limes' worth of juice, the scallions (if using), and the salt. Transfer to a bowl and loosely cover to keep warm.

5. In a large skillet over medium-high heat, heat the remaining 1 tablespoon of oil. Add the beef and seasoning and cook for 4 to 5 minutes, stirring occasionally, until the beef is no longer pink.

6. Divide the cauliflower among 4 bowls, top with the meat and avocado (if using), and serve.

Per Serving: Calories: 250; Total fat: 12g; Saturated fat: 4g; Sodium: 252mg; Carbohydrates: 9g; Fiber: 3g; Sugar: 3g; Protein: 26g

Walnut Pesto Beef Skewers

Dairy-Free, Gluten-Free, Nut-Free, No Added Sugar, Omega-3-Rich, Soy-Free
Prep time: 15 minutes, plus 30 minutes to marinate / **Cook time:** 20 minutes
Makes 8 skewers

Basil is considered a medicinal herb in the mint family, and its essential oils have been shown to reduce inflammation, protect against chronic disease, and act as an adaptogen, helping the body combat stress.

1 pound flank steak, cut into 1-inch pieces
¼ cup olive or avocado oil, divided
3 tablespoons red wine vinegar, divided
¾ teaspoon salt, divided
¼ teaspoon freshly ground black pepper
½ teaspoon red pepper flakes, divided (optional)

1 cup fresh basil
2 tablespoons chopped walnuts
1 garlic clove
1 tablespoon water
1 tablespoon nutritional yeast (optional)

1. In a large glass dish, combine the steak pieces, 1 tablespoon of oil, 1 tablespoon of vinegar, ½ teaspoon of salt, the black pepper, and ¼ teaspoon red pepper flakes (if using). Stir well to evenly coat, cover, and refrigerate for 30 minutes up to 1 hour to help tenderize the meat.

2. Heat a grill to medium-high heat and lightly oil the grates. Thread the beef on 8 skewers. Place on the grill and close the lid. Grill for about 8 minutes total, turning once or twice to prevent burning.

3. Puree the basil, remaining 2 tablespoons of vinegar, the walnuts, the garlic, water, remaining 3 tablespoons of oil, remaining ¼ teaspoon of salt, the nutritional yeast (if using), and the remaining ¼ teaspoon of red pepper (if using). Cool slightly, top with pesto, and serve.

VARIATION TIP: To skip the grill, place the skewers in a casserole dish and roast in a 450°F oven for 8 to 10 minutes.

Per Serving (2 skewers): Calories: 277; Total fat: 19g; Saturated fat: 5g; Sodium: 352mg; Carbohydrates: 1g; Fiber: 0g; Sugar: 0g; Protein: 25g

Garlic-Mustard Steak

Dairy-Free, Gluten-Free, No Added Sugar, Nut-Free, Soy-Free
Prep time: 10 minutes, plus 1 hour to marinate / **Cook time:** 10 minutes • **Serves 4**

If you haven't tried grass-fed beef, this is a good recipe to start with. Grass-fed beef has great flavor, but some cuts of meat can be a little tough. Marinating steak before cooking helps tenderize it. This recipe calls for pan-searing, but an outdoor grill works just as well. This goes great with Chipotle Sweet Potato and Cauliflower Soup (page 48) or Chickpea and Kale Salad (page 57).

¼ cup extra-virgin olive oil

¼ cup balsamic vinegar

2 tablespoons Dijon mustard

2 garlic cloves, minced

1 teaspoon chopped fresh rosemary

1 teaspoon salt

½ teaspoon freshly ground black pepper

4 (6-ounce) boneless grass-fed sirloin
   steaks, about ½ inch thick

1. In a shallow baking dish, whisk together the olive oil, vinegar, mustard, garlic, rosemary, salt, and pepper.

2. Add the steaks and turn them to coat well with the marinade. Cover and let the steaks marinate for 1 hour at room temperature or up to overnight in the refrigerator.

3. Heat a large cast-iron skillet over high heat.

4. Remove the steaks from the marinade and blot them with a paper towel to remove any excess marinade. Cook the steaks for 2 to 3 minutes on each side or until caramelized and nicely browned.

5. Let the steaks rest for 5 minutes before serving.

PREP TIP: The marinade can be made up to a week ahead and can also be used on lamb chops or chicken. Store leftover steak in the refrigerator for up to 5 days.

Per Serving: Calories: 480; Total fat: 31g; Saturated fat: 8g; Sodium: 390mg; Carbohydrates: 3g; Fiber: 0g; Sugar: 2g; Protein: 48g

Lamb-Stuffed Peppers

Dairy-Free, Gluten-Free, No Added Sugar, Nut-Free, Soy-Free, Vegetarian Option (see headnote)

Prep time: 20 minutes / **Cook time:** 1 hour • **Serves 6**

Stuffed peppers make a delightful meal—satisfying and delicious in a neat little package. The lovely thing about stuffed peppers is you can use a multitude of ingredients for the filling. So, if you don't like lamb, swap in other ground meats, such as beef, chicken, or turkey. Change up the spices, add tomatoes and more. Create a vegetarian version using cooked quinoa and lentils as a fantastic alternative.

1 onion, finely diced

2 tablespoons water, plus additional for cooking

1½ pounds ground lamb

1 cup grated zucchini (about 1 zucchini)

¼ cup fresh basil, minced

1 teaspoon salt

½ teaspoon black pepper

6 bell peppers, any color, seeded, ribbed, tops removed and reserved

1. Preheat the oven to 350°F.

2. In a large pan over medium heat, sauté the onion in the water for about 5 minutes, or until soft. Add the ground lamb and zucchini. Cook for 10 minutes, breaking up the meat with a spoon. Stir in the basil, salt, and pepper. Remove from the heat.

3. Fill a 9-by-12-inch casserole dish with 1½ inches of water.

4. Stuff each pepper with an equal amount of the lamb mixture and place the peppers in the dish. Cap each pepper with its reserved top.

5. Place the dish in the preheated oven and bake for 45 to 50 minutes.

VARIATION TIP: For a nightshade-free option, stuff the mixture into acorn squash instead.

Per Serving (1 pepper): Calories: 258; Total fat: 9g; Saturated fat: 3g; Sodium: 481mg; Carbohydrates: 10g; Fiber: 3g; Sugar: 6g; Protein: 34g

Herbed Lamb Zucchini Boats

Dairy-Free, Gluten-Free, No Added Sugar, Nut-Free, Soy-Free
Prep time: 15 minutes / **Cook time:** 40 minutes • **Serves 6**

Many herbs are delicate, tender, and easily bruised. Not rosemary. It's fragrant and robust, filled with calcium and iron, and contains compounds that reduce inflammation, help with digestion, and enhance memory.

2 garlic cloves

6 zucchini, ends trimmed, halved lengthwise

2 tablespoons olive oil

1 onion, finely diced

1 pound ground lamb

1 to 2 tablespoons fresh rosemary, minced

½ teaspoon salt

½ cup shredded Gruyère or aged white
    cheddar (optional)

1. Preheat the oven to 350°F. Line a baking sheet with parchment paper. Mince the garlic and set it aside for 10 minutes.

2. With a small spoon, gently hollow out about 1 inch of space along the length of the inside of the zucchini halves. Reserve the zucchini flesh.

3. In a large skillet on medium heat, heat the oil and sauté the onion for about 5 minutes, or until softened. Add the garlic and sauté for 1 to 2 minutes, until fragrant.

4. Add the zucchini flesh, ground lamb, rosemary, and salt. Cook for 10 minutes, breaking up the lamb with a spoon. Remove from the heat.

5. Place the zucchini hollow-side up on the baking sheet and fill each zucchini half with equal amounts of the lamb mixture. Sprinkle with cheese (if using).

6. Bake for 25 minutes, or until the lamb is fully cooked and the zucchini are tender.

Per Serving (2 boats): Calories: 186; Total fat: 6g; Saturated fat: 3g; Sodium: 272mg; Carbohydrates: 9g; Fiber: 3g; Sugar: 4g; Protein: 24g

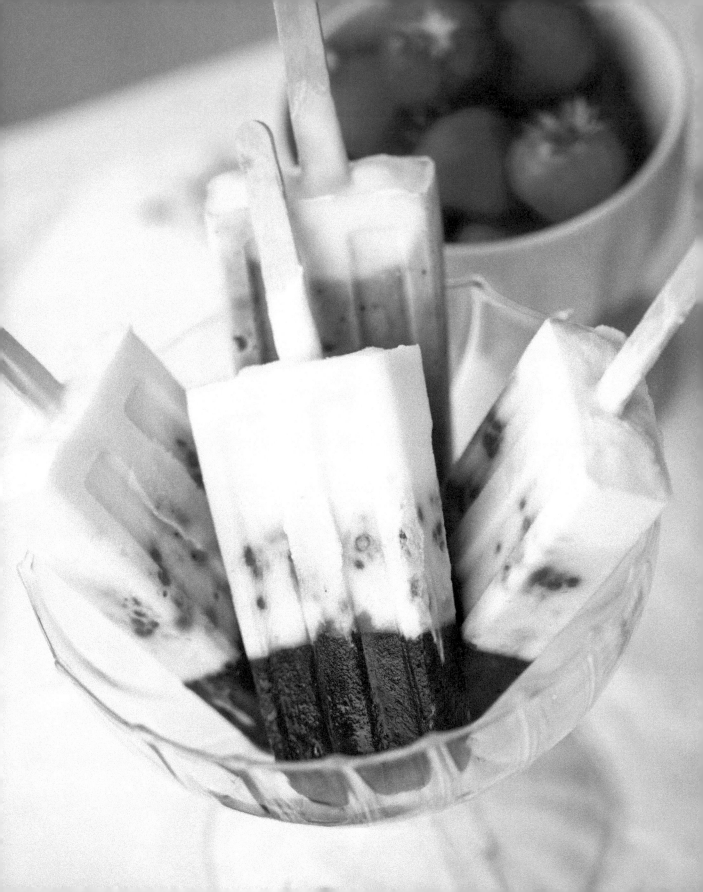

CHAPTER 8

DESSERT

Broiled Cinnamon Apple Crumble

Gluten-Free, Nut-Free, Soy-Free, Vegetarian
Prep time: 10 minutes / **Cook time:** 3 minutes • **Serves 4**

This recipe is a homage to delicious family apple pie from holiday get-togethers, without the work of figuring out a gluten-free crust. The tart Granny Smith apple slices are the perfect foundation for the honey-butter-cinnamon topping. Feel free to use dairy-free butter. Your body will thank you for skipping the cups of flour, sugar, and shortening found in traditional pie. These go fast, so consider doubling or tripling the recipe if you have a large crowd.

3 large Granny Smith apples, cored and sliced thick

2 tablespoons salted butter, melted

1 tablespoon honey

2 tablespoons oats, pulsed into crumbs or finely chopped

½ teaspoon cinnamon

1. Preheat the oven to broil. Line a baking sheet with parchment paper and arrange the apple slices in a single layer on the prepared sheet.

2. In a small bowl, mix the melted butter, honey, oats, and cinnamon. Spread the mixture onto each apple slice.

3. Broil for 2 to 3 minutes, until the topping becomes golden and caramelized. Transfer to a cooling rack, cool for 1 to 2 minutes, then enjoy warm.

VARIATION TIP: Replace the oats with almond flour to go grain-free. I also like to replace the honey with allulose to keep the sugar content even lower.

Per Serving: Calories: 167; Total fat: 6g; Saturated fat: 4g; Sodium: 47mg; Carbohydrates: 27g; Fiber: 5g; Sugar: 19g; Protein: 1g

Dark Chocolate Superfood Bark

Gluten-Free, Soy-Free, Vegan, Vegetarian
Prep time: 10 minutes, plus 15 minutes to chill / **Cook time:** 5 minutes • **Serves 16**

Cadmium and lead are heavy metals that are prevalent in the chocolate industry. Montezuma's Absolute Black Chocolate Bar (unsweetened), Trader Joe's Pound Plus 72% Cacao, and the Endangered Species Chocolate Strong+ Velvety Bar are all great-quality, low-heavy-metal choices.

16 ounces dark chocolate (70% cacao or above), broken into pieces
1 tablespoon sweetener of choice (allulose, maple syrup, honey, coconut sugar, etc.)
½ cup chopped nuts and seeds (cashews, almonds, pistachios, pumpkin seeds, etc.)
½ cup dried fruit (goji berries, candied ginger, cranberries, cherries, apricots, etc.)
1 handful coconut flakes
1 teaspoon sea salt

1. Line a baking sheet with parchment paper. Fill the bottom of a double boiler with 1 to 2 inches of water and reinsert the top pot. Or, place a medium glass bowl on top of the pot to act as a double boiler. Combine the chocolate and sweetener in the top pot/bowl. Bring the water to a simmer over medium-low heat and stir to encourage melting. Remove the chocolate from the heat as soon as most of the chocolate has melted, 4 to 5 minutes. Continue stirring until the chocolate is smooth.

2. Pour the chocolate evenly on the prepared baking sheet. Sprinkle the nuts, seeds, dried fruit, coconut flakes, and sea salt over the chocolate.

3. Refrigerate the baking sheet for 1 hour or freeze for 15 minutes. Once the bark has cooled completely and is hard, break it into pieces using your hands. Serve or refrigerate for up to 1 week or freeze for up to 1 month.

PREP TIP: To speed up the chocolate melting, microwave the chocolate in a glass bowl in 30-second intervals. Stir after each interval and remove as soon as most of the chocolate is melted.

Per Serving (1 ounce): Calories: 214; Total fat: 15g; Saturated fat: 8g; Sodium: 89mg; Carbohydrates: 18g; Fiber: 4g; Sugar: 10g; Protein: 3g

No-Bake Pumpkin Almond Butter Energy Balls

Dairy-Free, Gluten-Free, Omega-3-Rich, Soy-Free, Vegan, Vegetarian

Prep time: 10 minutes, plus 30 minutes to chill • **Makes 12 balls**

After learning of the sweetener allulose (first discovered and produced in Japan), its ability to act as an equal substitute for sugar in baking and cooking, and that most of it is eliminated in urine rather than metabolized by the body, I was sold. Recent research published in *Molecular Nutrition & Food Research* suggests allulose possesses anti-inflammatory properties and promotes the growth of beneficial bacteria in the gut.

½ cup canned pureed pumpkin (not pie filling)

⅓ cup creamy almond butter

3 tablespoons ground flaxseed

2 tablespoons allulose (or granule sweetener of choice)

1 teaspoon ground cinnamon

1. In a food processor, combine the pumpkin, almond butter, flaxseed, sweetener, and cinnamon and process until smooth. Alternatively, add all the ingredients to a medium bowl and manually mix. Chill the bowl in the refrigerator for 15 minutes.

2. Using a spoon or small scooper, scoop about a tablespoon of the mixture into your hands and roll into a ball. Repeat until all the dough is used.

3. Refrigerate in a sealed container for up to 2 weeks or freeze for up to 3 months.

VARIATION TIP: Replace the almond butter with sunflower or pumpkin seed butter for a nut-free option. You can add 2 tablespoons of mini chocolate chips for another variation.

Per Serving (1 ball): Calories: 56; Total fat: 4g; Saturated fat: 0g; Sodium: 3mg; Carbohydrates: 3g; Fiber: 2g; Sugar: 1g; Protein: 2g

Matcha Lime Coconut Ice Pops

Dairy-Free, Gluten-Free, Soy-Free, Vegan Option (see headnote)
Prep time: 10 minutes, plus 4 hours to chill • **Serves 6**

Matcha is an antioxidant powerhouse, so I'm always creating ways to incorporate more of it. In fact, matcha contains more polyphenols, or healthy bioactive substances, than cacao, coffee, and turmeric. Because chronic inflammation creates free radicals and induces oxidative stress in the body, antioxidant-rich foods and substances become even more important as we age and battle various forms of stress. To make this vegan, use vegan vanilla pea protein.

1 (14-ounce) can full-fat coconut milk

4 scoops vanilla protein powder (I prefer vanilla collagen peptides)

6 tablespoons granule sweetener of choice (I prefer allulose)

2 teaspoons matcha powder

Juice of 2 limes

1 scoop spirulina (optional)

1. In a blender, combine the coconut milk, protein powder, sweetener, matcha powder, lime juice, and spirulina (if using) and blend until smooth. Taste and adjust sweetness, lime, and matcha as desired.

2. Pour the mixture into ice pop molds and freeze for at least 4 hours. Allow to sit at room temperature for about 5 minutes before removing from molds.

VARIATION TIP: Not a fan of matcha but still want a boost in health-promoting flavonols? Replace the matcha with a low-cadmium/lead unsweetened cocoa powder (such as Ghirardelli 100% Cocoa or CocoaVia Cardio Health Dark Chocolate mix).

Per Serving (½ cup): Calories: 207; Total fat: 14g; Saturated fat: 13g; Sodium: 88mg; Carbohydrates: 10g; Fiber: 0g; Sugar: 0g; Protein: 13g

Carrot Cake Bites

Dairy-Free, Gluten-Free, No Added Sugar, Soy-Free, Vegetarian, Vegan Option (see tip)
Prep time: 10 minutes / **Cook time:** 10 minutes • **Makes** about 12 bites

My family's favorite treat, requested for every holiday and birthday, is carrot cake with cream cheese frosting. Unfortunately, traditional carrot cake, loaded with sugar, dairy, and refined flour, isn't exactly a health food, despite the carrots. My carrot cake bites are reminiscent of carrot cake, but with better-for-you ingredients.

1 cup quick-cooking oats, divided

1 large egg

¼ cup golden raisins, divided

2 tablespoons hot water

⅛ teaspoon salt

1 teaspoon cinnamon

½ cup packed finely shredded carrots

2 tablespoons coconut butter or manna, melted (optional)

1. Preheat the oven to 375°F. Line a baking sheet with parchment paper.

2. In a blender jar or small food processor, pulse ½ cup of the oats to make oat flour. Then add the egg, 2 tablespoons of golden raisins, the hot water, the salt, and the cinnamon. Pulse until well combined and egg is whisked.

3. Transfer the contents to a medium bowl and mix in the remaining ½ cup of oats, remaining 2 tablespoons of golden raisins, and the carrots.

4. Using a heaping tablespoon or 1-ounce scoop, scoop portions onto the prepared baking sheet, making about 12 bites. Bake for 10 to 12 minutes, until the cookies are golden and set.

5. Remove the carrot cake bites from the oven and let them cool slightly. Drizzle with the melted coconut butter (if using) and serve.

VARIATION TIP: To make these vegan, replace the eggs with flax eggs. Mix 5 tablespoons water with 2 tablespoons ground flaxseed. Stir well and let sit for at least 5 minutes to gel before using.

Per Serving: Calories: 147; Total fat: 3g; Saturated fat: 1g; Sodium: 107mg; Carbohydrates: 26g; Fiber: 4g; Sugar: 7g; Protein: 6g

Chocolate Avocado Pudding

Dairy-Free, Gluten-Free, Nut-Free, Soy-Free, Vegan
Prep time: 10 minutes, plus 1 hour to chill • **Makes about 2 cups**

Dates are an incredibly nutritious natural sweetener. They're rich in fiber, B vitamins, and important minerals such as calcium, iron, magnesium, and potassium. They make a great snack when stuffed with nut or seed butter and can amp up the nutrient factor in a wide variety of desserts. I use soft, caramel-like Medjool dates, but try any you like. If the dates are a little dry, soak them in warm water for 5 minutes before blending the pudding.

10 Medjool dates, pitted

2 avocados, halved and pitted

½ cup cacao powder

¾ cup unsweetened flax or plant-based milk, divided

1. In a food processor, combine the dates, avocados, cacao powder, and ½ cup of milk. Blend until smooth. If the pudding is too thick, add the remaining ¼ cup of milk and blend well.

2. Refrigerate for 1 hour before serving.

VARIATION TIP: To enhance the flavor, add vanilla extract, peppermint extract, ground cinnamon, ground ginger, or even a pinch of ground turmeric.

Per Serving (½ cup): Calories: 488; Total fat: 36g; Saturated fat: 2g; Sodium: 15mg; Carbohydrates: 48g; Fiber: 14g; Sugar: 28g; Protein: 6g

Blueberry-Yogurt Ice Pops

Dairy-Free Option, Gluten-Free, Nut-Free, Soy-Free, Vegan
Prep time: 15 minutes, plus 2 hours to freeze • **Serves 6**

Ice pops are one of those treats that many people tend to buy, but they are really very simple to make at home—and homemade versions don't have the artificial colors and flavors, or as much sugar. Ice pop molds are inexpensive and a great investment, but you can also make ice pops with paper cups and popsicle sticks. Making these is an excellent "cooking" activity for children—and a great way to get them to eat more produce.

1 cup fresh blueberries

Grated zest and juice of ½ lime, divided

1½ cups unsweetened yogurt or dairy-free alternative

2 tablespoons maple syrup, honey, or allulose

¼ teaspoon cinnamon

1. In a small bowl, mash the blueberries and add the lime zest. Divide the blueberry mixture among 6 ice pop molds.

2. In a medium bowl with an electric hand beater (or using a blender), blend together the yogurt, lime juice, sweetener, and cinnamon.

3. Pour the yogurt mixture into the ice pop molds over the blueberries.

4. Freeze for at least 2 hours, or until solid.

VARIATION TIP: In this recipe, I like to mash the blueberries so they still have a little texture. If you prefer them completely smooth, puree them in a blender before adding them to the molds. This recipe also works with a variety of fruit. If you aren't in the mood for berries, use peaches, apricots, nectarines, plums, figs, cherries, or kiwi. You can also add some chopped dark chocolate or dark chocolate chips for extra flavor and nutrition.

Per Serving: Calories: 186; Total fat: 14g; Saturated fat: 3g; Sodium: 37mg; Carbohydrates: 16g; Fiber: 2g; Sugar: 12g; Protein: 2g

Chocolate Chia Seed Pudding

Dairy-Free, Gluten-Free, Nut-Free, Vegan, Vegetarian
Prep time: 5 minutes, plus 5 hours to chill • **Serves 5**

This decadent chia seed pudding makes a nice treat, snack, or dessert any time of day. Naturally sweetened with just a touch of maple syrup, this recipe is high in fiber and anti-inflammatory omega-3 fatty acids, thanks to the chia seeds. It's also antioxidant-rich thanks to the cocoa. Feel free to adjust the amount of maple syrup to your preferred sweetness. I like to add 2 servings of chocolate protein powder for an extra bump in nutrition.

1½ cups unsweetened plant-based milk (I like flax)

¼ cup chia seeds

2 tablespoons unsweetened cocoa powder

2 tablespoons maple syrup, or 3 tablespoons allulose

1 teaspoon pure vanilla extract

1. In a medium bowl, whisk the milk, chia seeds, cocoa powder, maple syrup, and vanilla. The cocoa may take 1 to 2 minutes to incorporate; keep whisking until no lumps remain. Cover the bowl and refrigerate it for 30 minutes.

2. Remove the bowl from the refrigerator and stir the mixture. Refrigerate it again for another 30 minutes and then stir it again, to ensure the mixture sets evenly. Leave the bowl in the refrigerator for 4 or more hours, until the mixture has a thick, pudding-like consistency.

3. Serve immediately, refrigerate for up to 5 days, or freeze for up to 2 months. If frozen, thaw in the refrigerator for 3 to 5 hours before serving. If the pudding has become too thick, stir in 1 to 2 teaspoons of milk to thin as needed.

VARIATION TIP: Get creative with toppings: Try adding sliced strawberries, banana slices, coconut flakes, or chopped nuts.

Per Serving: Calories: 178; Total fat: 9g; Saturated fat: 1g; Sodium: 48mg; Carbohydrates: 21g; Fiber: 9g; Sugar: 8g; Protein: 7g

Almond Butter Freezer Fudge

Dairy-Free, Gluten-Free, Vegan, Vegetarian
Prep time: 5 minutes / **Cook time:** 5 minutes • **Makes 16 squares**

Traditional fudge is loaded with refined sugar and butter, but you won't find any of those potentially inflammatory ingredients here. Instead, treat yourself with satiating, healthy fats, some plant protein, and a touch of sweetness. A small square of this fudge is an awesome way to satisfy your sweet tooth in a more nutritious way.

¾ cup almond butter

⅓ cup coconut oil

¼ cup nonnutritive sweetener, such as allulose or monk fruit

¼ teaspoon salt

1. Line a 9-by-5-inch loaf pan with parchment paper.

2. In a small saucepan on low heat, combine the almond butter, coconut oil, sweetener, and salt. Warm gently for about 5 minutes, or until everything is incorporated.

3. Pour the fudge into the prepared pan, smoothing it evenly with a spatula, and refrigerate for 1 hour.

4. Slice the fudge into 16 squares and freeze in a sealed container for up to 3 months.

VARIATION TIP: For a nut-free version, use tahini or sunflower seed butter in place of the almond butter.

Per Serving (1 square): Calories: 123; Total fat: 11g; Saturated fat: 4g; Sodium: 38mg; Carbohydrates: 6g; Fiber: 1g; Sugar: 4g; Protein: 2g

Grain-Free Coconut Fruit Crisp

Dairy-Free, Gluten-Free, Vegan, Vegetarian
Prep time: 5 minutes / **Cook time:** 30 to 35 minutes • **Serves** 6

This fruit crisp recipe is incredibly versatile. Use a single type of fruit or a combination of many. And it's ideal for any bruised fruit past its prime. Basically, any fruit works—berries, plums, cherries, apples, peaches, nectarines, pears, apricots, mango, pineapple, you name it. I like to make fruit crisps as seasonal as possible, relying on what I find at local markets. Use antioxidant-rich fruit, protein-packed seeds and low sugar content to keep your palate satisfied and your body well fueled. You can even eat this for breakfast with a dollop of Greek or almond yogurt on top.

3 cups mixed fresh berries (raspberries, blueberries, blackberries, etc.)
¾ cup unsweetened shredded coconut

½ cup sunflower or pumpkin seeds
¼ cup granulated sugar or allulose
¼ cup coconut oil

1. Preheat the oven to 350°F.

2. Spread the fruit in a 9-inch square baking dish.

3. In a small bowl, mix the coconut, sunflower seeds, and sugar. Stir in the coconut oil and incorporate it throughout using your hands.

4. Crumble the topping over the fruit and bake for 30 to 35 minutes, or until the topping is golden and the fruit is bubbling.

VARIATION TIP: You can use any nut or seed in the topping. If they're larger nuts, such as almonds, pecans, or walnuts, give them a rough chop before mixing with the rest of the topping ingredients.

Per Serving: Calories: 379; Total fat: 29g; Saturated fat: 11g; Sodium: 9mg; Carbohydrates: 29g; Fiber: 10g; Sugar: 18g; Protein: 4g

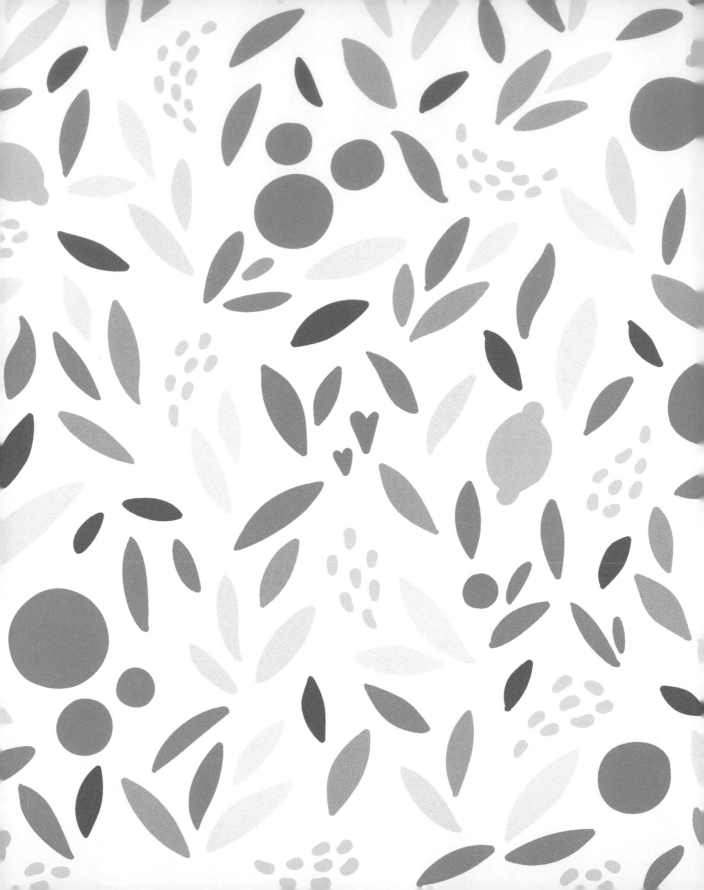

MEASUREMENT CONVERSIONS

Volume Equivalents	U.S. Standard	U.S. Standard (ounces)	Metric (approximate)
Liquid	2 tablespoons	1 fl. oz.	30 mL
	¼ cup	2 fl. oz.	60 mL
	½ cup	4 fl. oz.	120 mL
	1 cup	8 fl. oz.	240 mL
	1½ cups	12 fl. oz.	355 mL
	2 cups or 1 pint	16 fl. oz.	475 mL
	4 cups or 1 quart	32 fl. oz.	1 L
	1 gallon	128 fl. oz.	4 L
Dry	⅛ teaspoon		0.5 mL
	¼ teaspoon		1 mL
	½ teaspoon		2 mL
	¾ teaspoon		4 mL
	1 teaspoon		5 mL
	1 tablespoon		15 mL
	¼ cup		59 mL
	⅓ cup		79 mL
	½ cup		118 mL
	⅔ cup		156 mL
	¾ cup		177 mL
	1 cup		235 mL
	2 cups or 1 pint		475 mL
	3 cups		700 mL
	4 cups or 1 quart		1 L
	½ gallon		2 L
	1 gallon		4 L

Oven Temperatures

Fahrenheit	Celsius (approximate)
250°F	120°C
300°F	150°C
325°F	165°C
350°F	180°C
375°F	190°C
400°F	200°C
425°F	220°C
450°F	230°C

Weight Equivalents

U.S. Standard	Metric (approximate)
½ ounce	15 g
1 ounce	30 g
2 ounces	60 g
4 ounces	115 g
8 ounces	225 g
12 ounces	340 g
16 ounces or 1 pound	455 g

RESOURCES

FAVORITE PRODUCTS/BRANDS

Bob's Red Mill, BobsRedMill.com: For whole grains, flours and seed mixes. They offer a variety of products for those interested in organic, vegan, keto, paleo and more. I regularly use the gluten-free bean-based all-purpose baking flour, as well as their corn meal, tapioca flour, coconut flour, chickpea flour, almond flour, and more.

Con Olio, ConOlio.com: For high-quality olive oils.

Seasons, SeasonProducts.com: For seafood that is wild-caught, sustainable, and tinned in extra-virgin olive oil. Excellent source of omega-3 fatty acids and a convenient protein and fat option.

Thorne, Thorne.com: One of my favorite, reliable supplement companies.

Thrive Market, ThriveMarket.com: One-stop shop for healthy and organic products, delivered to your door.

Wild Planet, WildPlanetFoods.com: This is an excellent choice for skinless and boneless canned salmon. Regular and no-salt-added options available.

EDUCATION

Clear, James. *Atomic Habits*. New York: Random House, 2018.

Cole, Will. *The Inflammation Spectrum*. New York: Avery, 2019.

Consumer Lab, ConsumerLab.com: A valuable resource for information on supplements.

Huberman Lab. Andrew Huberman, HubermanLab.com: An excellent podcast for neurobiology and health science.

The Peter Attia Drive. Peter Attia, PeterAttiaMD.com: One of my favorite medical and longevity podcasts.

FoundMyFitness. Rhonda Patrick, PhD, FoundMyFitness.com: Another favorite podcast and website for longevity and health science.

Environmental Working Group. EWG.org: Consumer-friendly information about how to improve your environment and the effect of product choices on your health.

GI Map, DiagnosticSolutionsLab.com/tests/gi-map: A comprehensive tool to better understand your gut health.

Inside Tracker, InsideTracker.com: A home kit and online tracker of health metrics and data.

Nutrition by Natalie, NutritionByNatalie.com: My personal website with recipes, meal plans, virtual programs, articles, and more to help you optimize your health.

Omega Quant, OmegaQuant.com: My go-to test for identifying red blood cell omega-3 levels.

REFERENCES

Bella, Brita. "Researchers Find On-Off Switch for Inflammation Related to Overeating." June 30, 2020. medicalxpress.com/news/2020-06-on-off -inflammation-overeating.html.

Bordoni, Alessandra, Francesca Danesi, Dominique Dardevet, Didier Dupont, Aida S. Fernandez, Doreen Gillie, Claudia Nunes dos Santos et al. "Dairy Products and Inflammation: A Review of the Clinical Evidence." *Critical Reviews in Food Science and Nutrition* 57, no. 12 (August 13, 2017): 2497–2525. doi.org/10.1080/10408398.2014.967385.

Blair, Lisa, Kyle Porter, Binnaz Leblebicioglu, and Lisa Christiana. "Poor Sleep Quality and Associated Inflammation Predict Preterm Birth: Heightened Risk among African Americans." *Sleep* 38, no. 8 (August 2015): 1259–67. doi.org/10.5665/sleep.4904.

Bungau, Simona, Mohamed M. Abdel-Daim, Delia Mirela Tit, Esraa Ghanem, Shimpei Sato, Maiko Maruyama-Inoue, Shina Yamane, and Kazuaki Kadonosono. "Health Benefits of Polyphenols and Carotenoids in Age-Related Eye Diseases." *Oxidative Medicine and Cellular Longevity* 2019 (February 2019): 9783429. doi.org/10.1155/2019/9783429.

Casal, Susana, Ricardo Malheiro, Artur Sendas, Beatriz P. P. Oliveira, and José Alberto Pereira. "Olive Oil Stability under Deep-Frying Conditions." *Food and Chemical Toxicology* 48, no. 10 (October 2010): 2972–79. doi.org /10.1016/j.fct.2010.07.036.

Cerqueira, Érica, Daniel A. Marinho, Henrique P. Neiva, and Olga Lourenço. "Inflammatory Effects of High and Moderate Intensity Exercise: A Systematic Review." *Frontiers in Physiology* 10 (January 9, 2020): 1550. doi.org/10.3389 /fphys.2019.01550.

Choi, Yong Jun, Kyoung Hwa Ha, and Dae Jung Kim. "Exposure to Bisphenol A Is Directly Associated with Inflammation in Healthy Korean Adults." *Environmental Science and Pollution Research* 24 (2017): 284–90. doi.org /10.1007/s11356-016-7806-7.

Environmental Working Group. "EWG's Consumer Guide to Seafood." September 18, 2014. ewg.org/consumer-guides/ewgs-consumer-guide-seafood.

Gonzalez de Mejia, Elvira, Marco Vinicio Ramirez-Mares, and Sirima Puang-praphant. "Bioactive Components of Tea: Cancer, Inflammation and Behavior." *Brain, Behavior and Immunity* 23, no. 6 (August 2009): 721–31. doi.org/10.1016/j.bbi.2009.02.013.

Grzanna, Reinhard, Lars Lindmark, and Carmelita G. Frondoza. "Ginger: An Herbal Medicinal Product with Broad Anti-inflammatory Actions." *Journal of Medicinal Food* 8, no. 2. doi.org/10.1089/jmf.2005.8.125.

Han, Youngji, Eun-Young Kwon, and Myung-Sook Choi. "Anti-Diabetic Effects of Allulose in Diet-Induced Obese Mice via Regulation of mRNA Expression and Alteration of the Microbiome Composition." *Nutrients* 12, no. 7 (July 16, 2020): 2113. doi.org/10.3390/nu12072113.

Han, Youngji, Joon Yoon, and Myung-Sook Choi. "Tracing the Anti-inflammatory Mechanism/Triggers of D-Allulose: A Profile Study of Microbiome Composition and mRNA Expression in Diet-Induced Obese Mice." *Molecular Nutrition & Food Research* 65, no. 5. doi.org/10.1002/mnfr.201900982.

Harvard School of Public Health. *The Nutrition Source* (blog). "Kale." Accessed September 24, 2021. hsph.harvard.edu/nutritionsource/food-features/kale.

Irwin, Michael R., Richard Olmstead, and Judith E. Carroll. "Sleep Disturbance, Sleep Duration, and Inflammation: A Systematic Review and Meta-Analysis of Cohort Studies and Experimental Sleep Deprivation." *Biological Psychiatry* 80, no. 1 (July 2016): 40–52. doi.org/10.1016/j.biopsych.2015.05.014.

Lefevre, Michael, and Satya Jonnalagadda. "Effect of Whole Grains on Markers of Subclinical Inflammation." *Nutrition Reviews* 70, no. 7 (1 July 2012): 387–96. doi.org/10.1111/j.1753-4887.2012.00487.x.

Liu, Yun-Zi, Yun-Xia Wang, and Chun-Lei Jiang. "Inflammation: The Common Pathway of Stress-Related Diseases." *Frontiers in Human Neuroscience* 11 (2017): 316. doi.org/10.3389/fnhum.2017.00316.

Miękus, Natalia, Krystian Marszałek, Magdalena Podlacha, Aamir Iqbal, Czesław Puchalski, and Artur H. Świergiel. "Health Benefits of Plant-Derived Sulfur Compounds, Glucosinolates, and Organosulfur Compounds." *Molecules* 25, no. 17 (August 21, 2020): 3804. doi.org/10.3390/molecules25173804.

Navarro, Sandi L., Yvonne Schwarz, Xiaoling Song, Ching-Yun Wang, Chu Chen, Sabrina P. Trudo, Alan R. Kristal, Mario Kratz, David L. Eaton, and Johanna W. Lampe. "Cruciferous Vegetables Have Variable Effects on Biomarkers of Systemic Inflammation in a Randomized Controlled Trial in Healthy Young Adults." *Journal of Nutrition* 144, no. 11 (November 2014): 1850–57. doi.org/10.3945/jn.114.197434.

OmegaQuant (blog). "The Relationship between Omega-3 and Inflammation." January 17, 2019. omegaquant.com/what-do-omega-3s-do.

Owczarek, Danuta, Tomasz Rodacki, Renata Domagała-Rodacka, Dorota Cibor, and Tomasz Mach. "Diet and Nutritional Factors in Inflammatory Bowel Diseases." *World Journal of Gastroenterology* 22, no. 3 (January 21, 2016): 895–905. doi.org/10.3748/wjg.v22.i3.895.

Ruhee, Ruheea, and Katsuhiko Suzuki. "The Integrative Role of Sulforaphane in Preventing Inflammation, Oxidative Stress and Fatigue: A Review of a Potential Protective Phytochemical." *Antioxidants* 9, no. 6 (June 13, 2020): 521. doi.org/10.3390/antiox9060521.

Saltiel, Alan R., and Jerrold M. Olefsky. "Inflammatory Mechanisms Linking Obesity and Metabolic Disease." *Journal of Clinical Investigation* 127, no. 1 (January 3, 2017): 1–4. doi.org/10.1172/JCI92035.

Sears, Barry. "Anti-Inflammatory Diets." *Journal of the American College of Nutrition* 34 supplement 1 (September 2015): 14–21. doi.org/10.1080/07315724.2015.1080105.

Seitz, Adrienne. "The 11 Most Nutrient-Dense Foods on the Planet." Healthline. Last modified November 5, 2021. healthline.com/nutrition/11-most-nutrient-dense-foods-on-the-planet.

Simopoulos, A. P. "Omega-3 Fatty Acids in Health and Disease and in Growth and Development." *American Journal of Clinical Nutrition* 54, no. 3 (September 1991): 438–63. doi.org/10.1093/ajcn/54.3.438.

Wallace, Taylor C., Regan L. Bailey, Jeffrey B. Blumberg, Britt Burton-Freeman, C-y. Oliver Chen, Kristi M. Crowe-White, Adam Drewnowski, Shirin Hooshmand, Elizabeth Johnson, Richard Lewis et al. "Fruits, Vegetables, and Health: A Comprehensive Narrative, Umbrella Review of the Science and Recommendations for Enhanced Public Policy to Improve Intake." *Critical Reviews in Food Science and Nutrition* 60, no.13 (July 2019): 2174–2211. doi.org/10.1080/10408398.2019.1632258.

Wang, H. Joe et al. "Alcohol, Inflammation, and Gut-Liver-Brain Interactions in Tissue Damage and Disease Development." *World Journal of Gastroenterology* 16, no. 11 (March 21, 2010): 1304–13. doi.org/10.3748/wjg.v16.i11.1304.

Zhang, Hua, and Rong Tsao. "Dietary Polyphenols, Oxidative Stress and Antioxidant and Anti-inflammatory Effects." *Current Opinion in Food Science* 8 (April 2016): 33–42. doi.org/10.1016/j.cofs.2016.02.002.

INDEX

ACKNOWLEDGMENTS

I'm forever indebted to Joe Cho, who first advocated on my behalf to author a book. Thank you to my whole editorial team for helping make this cookbook the best it can be. I've worked with some brilliant practitioners, colleagues, and dietitians over the years, and I want to thank each one of you for inspiring me and helping me grow to where I am today.

Thank you to all my family and friends that have ever encouraged me, eaten my food, taste-tested recipes, given honest feedback, entertained my children while I worked, and supported me. I am humbled by your love and support. I now know that writing a book takes a village; thank you all for being a part of it. My cup runs over!

ABOUT THE AUTHOR

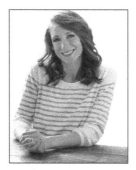

Natalie Butler, RDN, is a registered dietitian nutritionist, writer, speaker, and owner of Nutrition by Natalie, a private practice located in the Austin, Texas, area. Her main areas of interest and specialty are in nutrigenomics, longevity, gut health, and inflammatory conditions. Her practice offers consulting, recipe development, and medical review services for businesses, as well as online health programs and meal plans for individuals and families. Her professional experiences include Beautycounter, Whole Foods Market, Apple, Inc., Crossover Health, Healthline.com, MindBodyGreen.com, Head Health, Inc., Simple (an intermittent fasting app), local hospitals, and more.

Natalie loves spending time with her husband and three children cooking, gardening, tending to their chickens, and hiking in the great outdoors. You'll often find her exercising, geeking out over the latest science podcast, or reading a new health-related book. Natalie is a foodie at heart and loves most cuisines, but especially spicy Indian and Thai, and dark chocolate.

CPSIA information can be obtained
at www.ICGtesting.com
Printed in the USA
JSHW052048170722
27957JS00002B/2